How to
Heal Yourself
Using
Foot Acupressure
(Foot Reflexology)

by Michael Blate

ROUTLEDGE & KEGAN PAUL
London, Melbourne and Henley

This book is presented as a catalog and primer of techniques and other information that have been in continuous use throughout the Oriental and Western world for many years. While these techniques and information utilize a natural system within the body, there are no claims made for their effectiveness, even when properly used. These techniques and information are not an alternative to proper medical care and treatment, nor are they intended to supersede or replace any standard, Western first aid, emergency or medical techniques.

Illustrated by Michael Blate and Laurie Blate

First published in Great Britain in 1983
by Routledge & Kegan Paul plc
39 Store Street, London WC1E 7DD, England
464 St Kilda Road,
Melbourne, Victoria 3004, Australia
Broadway House, Newtown Road,
Henley-on-Thames, Oxon RG9 1EN, England
Printed in Great Britain by
Unwin Brothers Limited, The Gresham Press, Old Woking
Surrey GU22 9LH

British Library Cataloguing in Publication Data
Blate, Michael
How to Heal Yourself Using Foot Acupressure (Foot
    Reflexology)
1. Acupressure-therapeutic use. 2. Foot
1. Title
615. 8'22   RM 723 A27

ISBN 0–7102–0027–7

This book is for Andrea, because of <u>her</u> dedication...

"He who has subdued the mind will be the same in good times and bad. Grief and joy are but alternations of the mind. It is only when the mind is associated with the senses and the body that it is affected, agitated and modified."

Sri Sathya Sai Baba

CONTENTS

ACKNOWLEDGMENTS

The author wishes to thank and gratefully acknowledge the help and assistance of many members and friends of The G-Jo Institute. He is especially grateful to:

* Laurie Blate
* Al Fon
* Andrea Holly Gold
* Dick Knierim
* Sandy Pasquale
* Diane Ruby
* Barbara Sisson
* Jimmy Sullivan
* Sharon Tufaro
* Gail Watson
* Peggy Wells

WHAT IS THE G-JO INSTITUTE?

The G-Jo Institute is a not-for-profit natural health research and educational organization. It was informally organized in 1976 and incorporated in 1982. Its purpose is the development and dissemination of drugless "self-health" techniques.

G-Jo is a simplified form of acupuncture without needles (or "acupressure"). However, the scope of the G-Jo Institute has expanded far beyond its original purpose of the sharing of simple acupressure techniques.

It is our belief that it is the body-mind — and only the body-mind — which heals itself. For that reason, we now address ourselves to the entire spectrum of how to stimulate the innate self-healing mechanisms witihin the body-mind with simple, yet effective, self-health techniques from around the world.

For further information or catalogs about our publications, recordings, workshops and such, send a business-sized, self-addressed stamped envelope to:

THE G-JO INSTITUTE
DIVISION E
POST OFFICE BOX 8060
HOLLYWOOD, FLA. 33024
U.S.A.

HOW TO USE THIS MANUAL

1. Read the following information and familiarize yourself with the techniques described in this manual;

2. Look up your symptom or disorder in Section I (or, if you are not suffering any specific symptoms but wish to use foot acupressure as a general wellness and prevention technique, go immediately to step 4A);

3. Refer to those illustrated points detailed in Section II, suggested for that specific symptom you wish to treat. (Note: While most of the acupressure points have names that correspond to the symptom or bodily area each point controls, a few are simply referred to by a cross-reference listing — e.g., F-18, A-14, etc. These refer to unnamed points and are located by moving up or down the appropriate number line on the chart to the appropriate letter or horizontal line; this will correspond to the approximate location on your own foot);

4. Begin deeply pressing and "working" that approximate area on your own foot until you find one or several sensitive and tender spots that correspond to that area;

OR

-1-

4A. Deeply massage the entire foot until you discover all the tender spots — and then mark an "X" in the illustration of the feet that is found in the beginning of Section II (which may be photocopied, so as not to have to mark this book), for future reference and self-treatment;

5. Work the tender point(s) as deeply as you can manage for 30 seconds <u>or less</u> — they should become more tender (and may stay that way for up to several days) as self-treatment continues;

6. Rest for awhile afterwards;

7. Repeat self-treatment up to several times daily in the beginning of the process, but gradually reduce foot acupressure over the following period of several weeks;

8. Stop any obvious abuses (e.g., smoking, eating or drinking to excess, etc.) that may lead to — or aggravate — the problem...study as many natural health publications and techniques as you can... improve your diet...and take any other necessary steps to keep — or restore — pleasure, happiness and health to your life;

AVOID FOOT PRESSURE IF:

...you are a pregnant woman (especially beyond the third month of pregnancy);
...you are weakened, seriously ill or are taking regular medication for serious health problems (e.g., cancer, diabetes, etc.);
...you are a chronic heart patient (especially one who wears a pacemaker or other artificial energy-regulating device).

OVERVIEW

Foot acupressure — sometimes called "foot reflexology"
— is an ancient "self-health" technique that has been
widely used throughout the Orient for thousands of
years and which has become popular in the Western world
since the late 1960s. It is an easy-to-perform method
to restore health and wellness, or to bring yourself
symptomatic relief. This technique may be used by
anyone in normal health up to several times daily (see
instructions at the beginning of this book).

Foot acupressure points are thought to have both a
diagnostic and therapeutic value. If you have a
specific symptom — say, a headache or low back pain —
you may immediately turn to that specific symptom in
Section I of this manual and discover the appropriate
foot acupressure points to help relieve and "reverse"
(heal) that symptom.

Or, you may simply work on your entire foot —
pressing deeply until you discover tender spots — then
refer to Section II until you find the illustrations of
points which correspond to the tender areas you have
discovered. These may give you insight as to the state
of your internal organs and glands (each of these
points is thought to be somehow "connected" to a
so-called "reflex," which in turn leads to a specific
bodily area, organ or gland).

These points should be stimulated bilaterally —
that is, on both feet — unless otherwise stated. The
information about — and the location of the actual
site of — these points has been drawn from a number of
sources. Even so, their location on the illustrations

is _approximate_: The only true method for actually finding your own points is to press deeply — using up to 20 lbs. of pressure — until you contact a tender and sensitive "ouch point" in that approximate area of your own foot.

If you cannot find such a point in the approximate area, it usually means that you are either not pressing deeply enough, or the point is not going to be therapeutically effective. Nearly always, the most tender points are also the most effective for bringing relief and promoting healing. And for therapeutic purposes, use _only_ points which are tender to the touch. When they are no longer tender, discontinue their use.

Avoid any acupressure point that lies beneath a scar, mole, wart, etc. Wait about four hours after taking drugs, medications, alcohol (or other intoxicants) before applying foot acupressure. Wait about half an hour after taking a hot bath, doing strenuous labor or exercise, or eating a heavy meal before applying this technique. Other than that, acupressure may be used at any time.

HOW FOOT ACUPRESSURE WORKS

Foot acupressure is thought to work by affecting the flow of vital "life force" throughout the system. A complete healing network of energy-carrying channels is said to terminate in the feet. At one end of each channel is an organ, gland or other bodily area. At the other end — in the foot — is an acupressure point. Life force moves along these channels like electricity, to and from its various "terminals."

When life force — which we may call "bioenergy" — moves either too quickly or slowly along the channels, the organ or other bodily part malfunctions; symptoms and suffering soon follow. When a useful acupressure point is "triggered" and stimulated, it appears to at least temporarily restore a more normal or balanced flow of bioenergy.

ABUSE CAUSES SUFFERING

The process of disease and suffering is complex, yet the cause of most disease may be summed up in one word: Abuse. We abuse ourselves in many ways — wrong food and drink...unloving thoughts and emotions...work or home situations that are stress-filled and demeaning...the use of tobacco and/or recreational drugs — the list sometimes seems endless.

Surprisingly, most abuse is voluntary and self-inflicted. On one hand this reveals our own foolishness and self-destructive natures; yet on the other hand, this is a fortunate state of affairs — abuses which we inflict upon ourselves voluntarily can also be controlled, released or eliminated, if we so desire.

Neither acupressure — nor any other natural health technique — can be truly successful unless and until certain rules of healing are obeyed. These rules include the following:

1. To get well we must first <u>want</u> to get well
(this is the cardinal rule of healing — no healing
can occur unless and until we intend it to happen
and commit ourselves fully to the process);

2. We must discover — then release — the
self-abusive practices which keep us ill and
suffering; to speed healing, it is wise to replace
abusive practices with a better "healthstyle" —
right diet, moderate pleasures, and spiritual
self-development being of key importance;

3. We must be diligent in our efforts. Most adult
(chronic) suffering follows years of abuse, and what
takes years to develop cannot be cured in a matter
of days;

4. We must not become discouraged. The human
body-mind is a powerful self-healing mechanism that
is capable of "reversing" (healing) many of even the
most grievous ailments...as long as the above rules
are followed.

ABOUT "HEALING PHENOMENA"

Illness and suffering arise from abuses which are
somehow "stashed" and stored within the various organs
we are about to stimulate through foot acupressure.
The results of these abuses may be thought of as
"toxins" that will be purged from the system as the
healing process continues.
    It is not unusual for "healing phenomena" — brief
periods of cleansing — to occur during the course of
foot acupressure. This is a natural process — and a
beneficial one — so it should be understood and
appreciated.

Typical symptoms of cleansing include: Changes in bowel movements; headaches (especially at the beginning of self-therapy); digestive upsets; or similar ailments and malaise that might indicate "a flow of trash" being dumped into the system. Symptoms of cleansing might even include emotional distress (e.g., depression, bouts of anger, etc.). These symptoms — if they occur — should be mostly eliminated within several weeks of beginning foot acupressure.

However, unlike symptoms of illness, healing phenomena usually "feel right" — we do not sense that we are ill while "suffering" them... only cleansing ourselves.

NOTE TO READERS:

In the following pages, those words, acupressure points
or references which are fully CAPITALIZED are
considered to be the most important. Those words,
points or references which are underlined are considered of next importance.

ALSO: Following some of the acupressure point
names or numbers, you will find a question mark (?).
This should be taken as the author's suggestion —
neither confirmed nor denied by other published
healers, teachers or writers in the field of
acupressure — as to the most useful point(s) for the
target symptom or bodily area. When the question mark
procedes all acupressure points, this means the
author has not had first-hand experience with that
point or series of points for that symptom/bodily area,
but his suggestion is based upon his understanding of
the "Energy (acupuncture) Theory" and its applications.

SECTION I

SYMPTOMS, BODILY AREAS AND THE FOOT ACUPRESSURE POINTS WHICH AFFECT THEM:

Abdomen, lower
Abdomen, upper
Acne
Addiction
Adrenal glands
Alcohol, problems with
Allergies, non-specific
Anemia
Angina pectoris
Ankle
Anus
Apex (top of head)
Apoplexy (stroke)
Appendicitis
Appetite control
Appetite stimulation
Arm
Arthritis, minor
Asthma and asthmatic
    breathing, wheezing
Back, lower and/or upper
Baldness (alopecia)
Birth control
Bites, animal, human and
    insect
Bites, spider

Bladder, urinary
Bleeding gums
Boils, styes, carbuncles
Bones
Brain
Brainstem
Breasts
Breathing, difficult and
    labored
Bronchitis
Burns and scalds,
    including sunburn
Bursitis
Buttocks
Car sickness
Cataracts
"Charley horse"
Cheeks
Chemical burns
Chest
Cirrhosis
Clavicle (collarbone)
Coccyx
Colds and influenza
Colic, intestinal
Colitis

Colon
Congestion, sinus or
  nasal
Conjunctivitis (pink eye)
Constipation
Corns and bunions
Coronary thrombosis
Cough
Cramps, menstrual
Cramps and spasms,
  muscular
Cystitis
Dandruff
Deafness (sudden, acute)
Dental work
Depression (mental,
  emotional)
Dermatitis
Diabetes (diabetes
  mellitus)
Diaphragm
Diarrhea
Diverticulitis,
  diverticulosis
Dreaming, excessive
Duodenum
Dysentery
Dyspepsia
Dyspnea
Ear
Eczema
Edema
Elbow (including "tennis
  elbow")
Endocrine glands
Epiglottis
Epilepsy and epileptic
  seizures

Eustachian tubes
Eye
Face
Fatigue
Fever control centers
Fingers
Fits
Flatulence
Flu
Foot
Fractures
Frigidity (sexual)
Frostbite
Gallbladder
Gallstones
Gastritis (acid
  indigestion)
Gastrointestinal system
Genital weakness, pain
Genitourinary system
Gingivitis
Glands, swollen
Glaucoma
Gonorrhea
Gout
Hair
Hand
Hangover
Hay fever
Head
Headaches
Hearing difficulties
Heart
Heart attack, heart
  failure
Heel
Hemorrhage (bleeding)
Hemorrhoids (piles)

Hepatitis
Hernia (rupture)
Herpes simplex virus II
Herpes zoster virus
Hiccough (hiccups)
High blood pressure
Hip
Hives and rash
    (urticaria)
Hoarseness
Hunger control centers
Hyperactivity
Hypertension (high blood
    pressure)
Ileo-cecum
Hypoglycemia
Impetigo and eczema
Impotency (sexual)
Infection
Inflammations
Influenza
Insomnia
Intestinal problems
Intoxication
Itching; itchy skin
Jaundice
Jaw, lower
Jaw, upper
Kidneys
Kidney stones
Knee
Laryngitis
Larynx
Leg
Leg cramps (at night)
Liver
Lockjaw
Low blood sugar

Lumbago
Lungs
Lymph glands or nodes
Mastitis
Mastoid process
Menopause
Menstrual difficulties
Migraine
Mouth
Multiple sclerosis
Mumps
Muscles
Nasal congestion
    (catarrh)
Neck
Nephritis
Nerves
Nervousness
Neuralgia
Neurasthenia
Nightmares
Nose
Nosebleed (epistaxis)
Numbness
Occiput (back of head)
Ovaries
Pain control centers
Palate
Pancreas
Paralysis
Parasites, internal
Parathyroid glands
Parotid glands
Pelvis
Perineum
Periodontal problems
Peritonitis
Pharynx

Pineal gland
Pituitary gland
Pleurisy
Pneumonia
Prostate
Psoriasis
Rectum
Respiratory system
Retching
Rheumatism
Rhinitis
Scapula
Sciatica
Seasickness
Sexual drive
Sexual organs
Shingles
Shoulder
Sinusitis
Skin
Small intestine
Snoring
Solar plexus
Sores
Sore throat
Spasm, muscular
Spinal cord
Spleen
Sprains, muscular
Stomach
Stones, gallbladder
Stones, kidney or bladder
Strains, muscular
Styes
Swelling
Tennis elbow
Testicles, including
    crushed testicles

Tetanus (lockjaw)
Throat
Thymus gland
Thyroid (and parathyroid)
    gland
Tinnitus
Tongue
Tonsillitis
Tooth, teeth
Toothache
Tooth extraction,
    drilling, etc.
Torticollis (stiff neck)
Trachea
Travel sickness
"Traveler's diarrhea"
Trigeminal neuralgia
Ulcers, digestive
Ulcers, oral
Ulcers, skin
Ureters
Urethra
Urinary control centers
Uterus
Vaginitis
Varicose veins
Vertebrae, cervical
Vertebrae, lumbar
Vertebrae, sacral
Vertebrae, thoracic
Vertigo
Vitiligo
Vomiting and retching
Whiplash (neck injury)

ABDOMEN, LOWER (also see: Appendicitis; Peritonitis; etc.): The area between the navel and the pubic region. Organs found in this area include: The small intestine; colon (large intestine); urinary bladder; sexual/repro- ductive organs; etc.

Consider the following:

1. Pain that occurs throughout the entire abdomen (lower and upper) that is not localized nor extreme (a simple "bellyache") is probably from wrong food, constipation, etc;

2. Pain that occurs first at/near the navel, then shifts to the lower right quarter of the abdomen may be appendicitis;

3. Pain that is severe, cramplike and comes/goes, plus recurrent vomiting, abdominal distention, being gas-bound and constipated may indicate complete or (if there is diarrhea) partial blockage of the small intestine (esp. if pain centers at/near navel and if you have had an abdominal operation in the past);

4. Pain below the navel that is not too severe and is accompanied by distention, with difficulty in passing gas as well as difficulty in moving bowels (passing small, frequent stools, if any) may indicate partial/complete blockage of the colon/large intestine;

5. If you are a woman suffering pain in the lower right or left quarters of the abdomen that is sudden, severe and often accompanied by nausea and vomiting, it may be due to problems in the ovary, especially a twisted ovarian cyst;

continued next page...

6. Severe pain in the lower abdomen that gradually moves upward to the right upper quarter and stomach, increasing in intensity without relief (and with abdomen becoming hard) may be a symptom of peritonitis;

7. Frequently recurring pain that is relieved by passing gas, stools and especially if also accompanied by nausea, diarrhea, headaches, etc., may indicate colitis, pre-colitis or irritable colon;

8. Any lump in the groin or navel area, with or without pain, may indicate a hernia;

9. There are a number of other possibilities — intestinal flu, allergic reactions, poisoning, etc. — which might be considered;

If symptoms are not relieved by the following techniques, do the following:

1. Try each of the other sections listed for the above symptoms (e.g., Appendicitis, Gastrointestinal system, etc.) that most closely matches your symptoms;

2. If you still get no relief, avoid all foods and take only small amounts of water (or ice chips);

3. Get medical attention immediately.

Foot points: Appendix; Colon (all); Ileo-cecum; rear half of foot.

ABDOMEN, UPPER (also see: Small intestine; Stomach; etc.): The area between the diaphragm and the navel.

Included in this central portion of the body are: The liver; gallbladder; stomach; spleen; pancreas; small intestine; kidneys; adrenals; etc.

Pain/discomfort in the upper abdomen may indicate:

continued next page...

1. Simple indigestion — especially if the symptoms include: Nausea; heartburn; distention; a feeling of fullness; belching and/or flatulence; or any other similar symptoms which develop during or after a meal;

2. Gallbladder disorder — especially if the discomfort is located in the upper right quarter of the abdomen;

3. Pancreatitis (or other disorders of the pancreas) — especially if there is severe pain centering at/near the stomach, but extending to the back and chest and relieved by sitting up;

4. Heart attack, heart failure — which, in the beginning stages, is confused by some people with acute indigestion, etc.

As with disorders of the lower abdomen, there are many possible causes of distress. Follow the same rules as for problems in that region (see Abdomen, lower);

Foot points: Middle third of foot plus corresponding bodily parts.

ACNE (also see: Allergies, non-specific; Skin; etc.): Eruptions on the face, chest, back, etc. Acne is thought to arise from imbalance within the lungs, colon, kidneys and urinary bladder by traditional Oriental therapists. (Note: Acne tends to worsen during winter, to improve during summer, but excessively hot and/or humid weather may trigger an attack, as may the time just before, during and/or after menses).

Foot points: Lungs; Kidneys; plus corresponding bodily areas.

-15-

ADDICTION (to alcohol, drugs, tobacco, etc. — also
see: Alcohol, problems associated with; INTOXICATION;
etc.): Marked emotional or psychophysical dependence on
a substance — usually destructive — which is beyond
voluntary control. In traditional Oriental theory,
dependency and addiction are considered disorders
primarily of the spleen, pancreas and stomach ("Earth"
organs).

Foot points: (?) Lungs; Liver; Stomach; Spleen;
Pancreas.

ADRENAL GLANDS (also see: Endocrine glands;
Hypoglycemia; Kidneys; etc.): Endocrine glands are
found just above the kidneys; they are responsible for
the production of adrenaline (epinephrine) and numerous
other steroid hormones. Any self-treatment of these
glands should be done with caution and restraint.
    The adrenals are key glands in regulating bodily
reactions to stress and fear; their malfunctioning may
result in allergies, hypoglycemia, arthritis, asthma,
etc.

Foot points: Adrenals; Kidneys.

ALCOHOL, PROBLEMS ASSOCIATED WITH (also see:
Cirrhosis; INTOXICATION; etc.): Studies show that
females have a much lower tolerance for alcohol than
males.

Foot points: Liver; Spleen; Pancreas.

ALLERGIES, non-specific (also see: Other symptoms associated with allergies): A repeated bodily reaction upon exposure to an allergenic substance such as wood, feathers, etc.

"Unusual" or "hidden" symptoms of allergy may include: Insomnia; excessive perspiration; restlessness; increased sense of smell; depression; abnormal pulse and many other seemingly unrelated phenomena.

Allergies are generally not cured but rather are greatly reduced by proper "healthstyle." Each person has at least several foods/substances to which he is allergic. Food allergies, at least, appear to come in "degrees" (or "layers") so that after the most offensive abusive allergen is dropped or eliminated from the diet, the allergy(ies) next in "strength" begin exerting their influence. At the root of each allergy is thought to be the emotion of _fear_ controlled by the kidneys and adrenal glands.

Foot points: Appendix; Ileo-cecum; Adrenals.

ANEMIA (iron-deficiency type): A deficiency of red blood cells that is difficult — perhaps dangerous — to self-diagnose. Because internal bleeding (or such blood disorders as leukemia) may be responsible for this symptom, seek medical advice if anemia is suspected.

Foot points: Elbow; Liver; Thyroid; Intestine, small; Spleen; Colon.

ANGINA PECTORIS (also see: Chest; Heart; Heart attack, heart failure; Pain control centers; etc.): Deep spasmodic pain often radiating to the left arm and shoulder. It is often triggered by an emotionally or physically taxing experience. Get medical help immediately. Except in emergency, no pressure point stimulation should be used when regular daily medication is being taken; also, except when professional help is not available, self-treatment of heart disorders should be avoided (angina is the pain associated with coronary heart disease).

Angina is characterized by a pain (usually) in the center of the chest which also triggers a sense of fear or foreboding — a sense of warning that commands the sufferer to immediately stop what he is doing.

Angina responds quickly to rest. If the pain continues for longer than 15 minutes after relaxing, the pain is probably not angina.

Foot points: Heart.

ANKLE (also see: Foot; Sprains, muscular; Strains, muscular; etc.): For any injury to this joint, quickly remove shoe and stocking, since swelling tends to be rapid.

Foot points: Ankle; Foot, feet.

ANUS (also see: Colon; Gastrointestinal system; Hemorrhoids; Rectum; etc.): Lowest point of the rectum and termination of the alimentary canal. Common symptoms include: Hemorrhoids; prolapse (dropping or drooping of wall of colon through the anus); rectal itch; etc.

continued next page...

-18-

Possible causes of anal itch include: Rectal disorders (hemorrhoids, etc.); pinworms (or similar parasites); allergies; various diseases (e.g., diabetes, venereal herpes simplex virus, jaundice, uremia, etc.); infection from fecal matter; worms, internal parasites.

Foot points: Rectum; Prostate (females, also).

APEX (top) of Head (also see: Head; etc.): For pain or other symptoms in this area.

Foot points: Brain.

APOPLEXY (stroke): The result of a blood clot or hemorrhage to the brain or a major organ.
   While nearly all strokes are accompanied by some disability — usually paralysis, etc. — it is important to remember that much can be done to restore full/nearly full recovery. Aside from the following acupressure points, other "alternative" methods (such as acupuncture done with needles) are also available.

Foot points: Liver; Pituitary.

APPENDICITIS (also see: Abdomen, lower; etc.): An inflammation of the appendix, located below and slightly to the right of the navel. This may be a serious problem; there is the possibility of the appendix rupturing. Get medical help immediately.
   Many other problems may mimic appendicitis, such as: Stones/infection in the urinary tract (esp. in the ureter); ileitis; ovarian cyst in a female; etc.

Foot points: Appendix; Colon, ascending.

APPETITE CONTROL: See HUNGER CONTROL CENTERS.

APPETITE STIMULATION: To help improve and stimulate
the desire and hunger for food. Chronic loss of
appetite may produce anorexia nervosa, a potentially
dangerous condition of self-starvation (common
especially among weight-conscious women and those who
have successfully lost a substantial amount of extra
weight). Get professional help for this condition.

Foot points: (?) Stomach; Gallbladder; Liver.

ARM (also see: Elbow; Hand; Shoulder): Including both
the arm and armpit. There are several (potentially)
serious problems that can happen to the arm. Among
them are:

    1. Arterial blockage — characterized by:
Sudden coldness, tingling and/or numbness
developing in the arm, followed by severe pain;
blue or mottled patches developing on the skin,
etc.;
    2. Fracture — characterized by: Sudden, sharp
pain, especially upon movement of the affected
arm;
    3. Thrombophlebitis (clot lodged in a vein) —
characterized by: Warming of the skin at/near
affected site; swelling; (esp. sudden) deep,
aching pain; etc.
    4. Symptom of heart disease (e.g., angina
pectoris), impending/progressing heart attack,
etc. — especially if pain radiates down the
left arm.

continued next page...

If you notice any of the above symptoms, get medical help immediately.

Other less serious problems may include: Strains; sprains of the elbow, wrist, shoulder; inflammation; etc.

Foot points: Arm.

ARTHRITIS, minor (acute): A catchall name for a number of symptoms that manifest themselves primarily as inflammation of the joints; it is suffered mostly by women. There are numerous self-help techniques detailed in this author's HOW TO RELIEVE ARTHRITIS WITH ACUGENICS (available through the G-Jo Institute).

Foot points: Use points for affected bodily areas.

ASTHMA and ASTHMATIC BREATHING, WHEEZING, ETC. (also see: Dyspnea; etc.): Massive narrowing and constriction of the air passages in the throat. Its symptoms include coughing, wheezing, panic, etc. Get medical help immediately.

Most studies agree that an asthmatic's parents are an important root in the disorder — either overly protective or too unconcerned. Any therapy should take this into consideration.

Foot points: Lungs; Adrenals.

BACK, LOWER and/or UPPER (also see: Lumbago; Pain control centers; Sciatica; etc.): Backache — especially lower backache — is one of modern man's most common symptoms.

"Common" low back pain is often as much a disorder of the abdominal (bulky, unsophisticated lower trunk) muscles as one of the lower back. Back pain may also result from a number of more serious disorders (e.g., kidney stones, etc.) — if symptoms persist, see your doctor.

Foot points: Vertebrae (all); Coccyx.

BALDNESS (alopecia): Often caused by excess male hormones in system. Generally hair loss is normal, as is hair regeneration; life of a strand of hair is about three years. Imbalanced or malfunctioning liver and kidneys are considered the organs most responsible for hair loss (and regeneration). Where there is baldness in front, it may be a symptom of excess fruits, liquids or intestinal disorders; when baldness is mostly on top, excess animal protein; when baldness occurs in back, excess drugs or chemicals; when baldness occurs at temples, may indicate excess sweets, drugs.

Foot points: Thyroid; Kidneys; Lungs.

BIRTH CONTROL: There are a number of natural methods to promote or prevent pregnancy. However, they should only be used with discretion and only when willing to accept the consequences of failure. The various acupressure points that may be useful include:

Foot points: Stimulate Kidneys to increase fertility.

-22-

BITES, ANIMAL, HUMAN AND INSECT: If you are
bitten by a wild creature, there is a possibility of
rabies, especially if the bite is from a skunk,
squirrel, raccoon or other small mammal. Try capturing
the animal alive for observation in captivity. Killing
the animal is less desirable; but if done, keep the
head refrigerated until it can be tested in a
laboratory.

There are three possible states for a rabid animal
to be in:
1. Furiously vicious, foaming at the mouth, etc.;
2. Sluggish-to-paralyzed;
3. Behaving "peculiarly" — that is, without normal
fear of humans, aggressive behavior, daylight
activity in ordinarily nocturnal creatures (e.g.,
bats, foxes, etc.).

Bites from animals in the above states call for
immediate attention.

Foot points: Corresponding bodily area points.

BITES, SPIDER: Many spiders are somewhat poisonous,
but the two most common truly poisonous spiders are the
(female) black widow and the brown household (or brown
recluse).

Symptoms include pain, abdominal cramps, sometimes
paralysis, tenderness, redness, and swelling around the
bitten area. Get medical help immediately.

Foot points: Corresponding bodily area points.

BLADDER, URINARY (also see: STONES, KIDNEY OR BLADDER; Cystitis; Genitourinary system; Urinary control centers;): The organ of accumulation for urine. In traditional Oriental theory, this is considered one of the twelve principal organs and is paired with the kidneys. As such, it helps "control" fear, sexual drive, caution, etc. (For more in-depth techniques for healing this organ, see this author's THE NATURAL HEALER'S ACUPRESSURE HANDBOOK, VOLUME II.)

Foot points: Bladder (urinary); Kidneys.

BLEEDING GUMS: See Gingivitis.

BOILS, STYES, CARBUNCLES (also see: SKIN; "Sores"; etc.): Localized "staph" infections of varying degrees of severity. They are often found around the eyes (styes), neck, back, or buttocks. Often associated with disorders in the genitourinary system.

Foot points: Use corresponding bodily area points.

BONES (also see: Fractures; etc.): Bones are related to kidneys, according to Oriental therapists. Any bone disorders may also indicate kidney imbalances.

Foot points: Kidneys; Adrenals; corresponding bodily area points.

BRAIN (also see: Brainstem; Nerves; etc.): Primary portion of the central nervous system.

Foot points: Brain; Pituitary; Pineal.

BRAINSTEM (also see: BRAIN; etc.): Central part of the brain.

Foot points: Brain.

BREASTS: (also see: Mastitis; etc.): Intimately related to the stomach and/or liver in Oriental literature.

Foot points: Stomach; Breast.

BREATHING, Difficult and Labored: See Dyspnea.

BRONCHITIS (also see: Chest; Cough; Respiratory system; Throat; etc.): An inflammation of the bronchial "tree" whose symptoms include: Fever, pains in the back and muscles, headache, etc.

Foot points: Adrenals; Colon; Lungs.

BURNS and SCALDS, including sunburn: There are different types of burns as well as degrees of severity:
    a. Thermal (heat) burns: Immerse the area in a slush of freshwater ice and water, or let cold water flow from faucet onto burned area (up to 15 minutes);

continued next page...

b. Chemical burns: Flush chemicals from the tissue immediately;

c. Sunburn: See below.

Minor (first-degree burns) cause redness and minor swelling to the affected site. More serious burns manifest blisters and additional swelling (second-degree) or leave the skin looking white or charred (third degree — the worst kind of burn). Third-degree burns may not be as painful as the less serious form because of underlying nerve damage. If a limb has been burned, keep it elevated. In more serious burns, shock is likely.

For more serious burns, drink plenty of water with a little salt and baking soda added to help replace the salty fluids of the body and reduce the possibility of shock. Do not apply ointments or pastes such as baking soda in the case of a severe burn; they will only have to be scraped off at a hospital or burn center. Get medical help immediately.

Foot points: Corresponding bodily area points.

BURSITIS (also see affected areas, such as Shoulder, etc.): An inflammation between moving joints. Immobilize the affected extremity (generally the arm or shoulder).

Foot points: Shoulder; or corresponding bodily area point.

BUTTOCKS (also see: Hip; etc.):

Foot points: Hip; Kidneys; Rectum; Vertebrae, sacral.

CAR SICKNESS: See Seasickness; Travel sickness; etc.

CATARACTS (also see: Eyes; etc.): Partial or complete opacity of the eye lens or its capsule. Often related to diabetes, excess galactose (from milk), fatty acid intolerance, irradiation, drugs, etc. May be related a liver disorder, according to Oriental therapists.

Foot points: Eye; Liver; Gallbladder.

"CHARLEY HORSE": See CRAMPS and SPASMS, MUS-CULAR; LEG; STRAINS, MUSCULAR.

CHEEKS (also see: Face; Head; Mouth; etc.):

Foot points: Ear; Eye; Tongue.

CHEMICAL BURNS: See Burns and Scalds.

CHEST (including Pain, Intercostal Neuralgia, etc. — also see: Breasts; Heart; Heart attack; Lungs; Respiratory system; etc.): Common name for the thorax, located between the diaphragm and neck. Any recurring pain or heaviness in this area — especially any discomfort that seems to radiate down the left arm — should receive prompt medical attention because it might indicate a serious heart condition.
   Organs within the chest (thorax) include: The lungs; heart; breathing/air passages; (and within the ribcage are also: The spleen; pancreas; upper portions of the stomach and liver; diaphragm; etc.).

continued next page...

Pain/discomfort in the chest area may have many causes. Among the most serious of them are the following:

1. Angina (angina pectoris) — especially if it is characterized by a choking or suffocating pain (usually) in the center of the chest which also triggers a sense of fear or foreboding and which generally arises after physical exertion. Angina pains will generally cease within 15 minutes of stopping and resting;

2. Heart attack, heart failure (cardiac arrest) — especially if the pain ranges from moderate pressure to crushing or vise-like and does not respond to rest. Other common symptoms include: Grave anxiety (with a feeling death is near); shortness of breath; vomiting and retching; belching; face turning gray/ashen, especially with clammy perspiration; etc. (Note: It is probably not a heart attack — but may be angina — if pain: Is below and to the left of the nipple; stays completely on the left side; is sharp/cutting rather than a dull/squeezing sensation; comes/goes or is relieved by lying down/lasts for only several minutes);

3. Rupture of an aortic aneurysm — often mimics heart attack/heart failure;

4. Pneumothorax — especially if there is sharp pain extending from shoulder to abdomen, breathing difficulty, and follows recent disorder of the chest area.

Other less serious/less common problems may include: Pleurisy; injury to the ribs or their muscles (especially if there is a dull, gnawing ache and/or if moving or staying in a certain position is painful); problems in the esophagus; lung disorders (e.g., abscesses, aerophagia — the swallowing of air — pneumonia, colds, etc.); indigestion; hiatal hernia; etc.

Foot points: Breast; Lungs; Heart.

CIRRHOSIS (of the liver — also see: LIVER; etc.): A destructive (atrophying) disease of the liver often associated with over-consumption of alcohol. Complete (vs. incomplete) protein is vital for regeneration.

Foot points: (?) Liver; Gallbladder; Spleen; Pancreas.

CLAVICLE (collarbone — also see: Fractures; etc.): The long bone(s) at the top of the chest stretching across to the tips of the shoulders. The following acupressure points may be helpful following fractures, etc.

Foot points: Neck; Shoulder.

COCCYX: The small, bony protrusion at the bottom of the spine, commonly called the "tailbone."

Foot points: Coccyx; Vertebrae, sacral;

COLDS and INFLUENZA (also see accompanying symptoms such as: Cough; Headaches; Nasal congestion; etc.): The word "colds" has been applied to many symptoms that come together and last for about seven days; an upper respiratory infection.
    Symptoms of colds and influenza include fever, cough, dull aches and pains, nasal congestion (catarrh), etc.

Foot points: Lungs; Adrenals.

COLIC, INTESTINAL (also see: Abdomen, lower, upper; Colon; Gastrointestinal system; Small intestine; etc.): Spasmodic abdominal pain, due to obstruction, twisting or cramping in the smooth muscles. In infants may be due to swallowing air, overfeeding, milk too rich, intestinal allergies, emotional distress, etc., and may be expressed by symptoms such as red face, irritability, pulling knees up to stomach, etc.

Foot points: Colon (all); Liver; Stomach.

COLITIS (also see: Abdomen, lower; Gastrointestinal system, etc.): A usually chronic inflammation of the colon. Often associated with buried anger (a liver disorder) and resentment (lungs) by Oriental therapists. Some form of psychotherapy may be helpful in conjunction with the following techniques. Chronic colitis (which involves tissue changes in the colon) requires professional attention.

Foot points: Colon (all); Intestine, small; Liver.

COLON (LARGE INTESTINE, including ascending, transverse, descending and sigmoid colon — also see: Abdomen, lower; Colic, intestinal; COLITIS; Constipation; Diarrhea; GASTROINTESTINAL SYSTEM; etc.): That part of the gastrointestinal tract beginning with the ileo-cecum and ending at the sigmoid flexure. Considered one of the twelve principal organs in traditional Oriental theory, it is thought to be paired with the lungs. It has a number of diverse functions. (For more in-depth techniques for healing this organ, see this author's THE NATURAL HEALER'S ACUPRESSURE HANDBOOK, VOLUME II.)

Foot points: Colon (all); Liver; Lungs.

CONGESTION, SINUS OR NASAL: See Nasal congestion (catarrh).

CONJUNCTIVITIS (pink eye — also see: Eye; Liver): An inflammation and reddening of the membrane (conjunctiva) covering the front of the eye. It is generally considered a liver disorder by Oriental therapists.

Foot points: Eye; Liver.

CONSTIPATION (costiveness — also see: Gastrointestinal system): A condition wherein the bowels move infrequently or with great difficulty. It may be chronic or acute and is associated with a great number of physical or mental disturbances.
Constipation is generally associated with liver and/or kidney disorders by traditional Oriental therapists.
There are numerous symptoms of constipation — surprisingly, the failure to move bowels regularly   is not necessarily one of them (constipated people may have several bowel movements daily). Included are the following:
    1. Hemorrhoids, colitis or similar bowel disorders;
    2. Fatigue, irritability, etc.;
    3. Feeling of heaviness and/or fullness;
    4. Swollen lips (esp. lower lip);
    5. Foul breath, body odors;
    6. Gas/flatulence (chronic, not occasional);
    7. Strong-smelling urine;
    8. Feeling of fullness, heaviness or being "loaded";
    9. Chronic feelings of grief, depression, anxiety, etc.;
  10. Skin eruptions, pimples, blackheads, etc.;

continued next page...

Foot points: Thyroid; Liver; Colon, ascending-to-transverse-to-descending-to-rectum (in that order and direction!); Kidneys.

CORNS and BUNIONS (also see: Foot; Skin; etc.): Horny layers of growth upon the skin which project inwards as well as outwards, usually caused by friction (corns); or a swelling (bursa) especially around or near the joint of the big toe upon the foot. Generally caused by ill-fitting shoes, either too pointed and/or too short and/or with heels that are too high.

Foot points: Massage exact point on opposite foot.

CORONARY THROMBOSIS: (Myocardial infarction — also see: HEART; Heart attack, heart failure; etc.): Damage to (part of) the heart muscle from a clot of blood, most generally lodged in an artery supplying the heart. Symptoms often include: A feeling of oppression in the chest; pain beneath the sternum (breastbone), often described as squeezing, pressing or constricting; dyspnea (labored breathing) with or without pain; skin that is pale, cold and moist; etc. Any of these symptoms — especially where there is a history of heart problems — require immediate medical attention.
    The following techniques are emergency remedies only and do not replace proper medical care.

Foot points: (?) Heart.

COUGH (also see: Respiratory system; Bronchitis; Colds and influenza, etc.): This condition may arise from a number of causes and be symptomatic of many ailments. (Note: Medical attention is important for chronic coughs or bloody coughs — especially those with no apparent reason).

Foot points: Lungs.

CRAMPS, MENSTRUAL: See Menstrual difficulties.

CRAMPS and SPASMS, MUSCULAR (also see: Leg; Pain control centers; etc.): Painful, involuntary spasms of muscles anywhere in the body, but especially of the leg or foot during sleep.

Foot points: (?) Foot, feet; Knee; Hip; Liver.

CYSTITIS (also see: Bladder; Genitourinary system; etc.): An inflammation of the bladder. Often there is a need to urinate, but only a few drops are passed, generally accompanied by a cutting, burning sensation.

Foot points: Kidneys; Bladder (urinary); Sex organs.

DANDRUFF (seborrheic dermatitis — also see:
DERMATITIS; SKIN; HAIR; etc.): Falling, greasy scales
of skin from the scalp, usually accompanied by itching
and possibly lesions. It may affect the eyebrows as
well.

Foot points: See DERMATITIS.

DEAFNESS, Sudden; Acute (also see: Ear; Hearing
difficulties; etc.): Total or partial loss of hearing,
often associated with inflammation or growths within
the ear canal, but may stem from a number of causes.
Get medical help immediately.

Foot points: See EAR.

DENTAL WORK (also see: Toothache; Tooth, teeth; etc.):
The following acupressure points may be helpful for
those who cannot have or choose not to have anesthesia
for dental work. Stimulate regularly during dental
work.

Foot points: Colon; Tooth, teeth.

DEPRESSION, MENTAL/EMOTIONAL (also see: FATIGUE;
Hypoglycemia; etc.): Extreme sadness, melancholy or
dejection which is unrealistic and not in proportion to
one's actual circumstances. Often diet-related,
according to traditional Oriental therapists, and has
its roots in the liver, lungs and heart.

continued next page...

In traditional theory, depression is both a cause and effect (symptom) of disturbed blood chemistry. It is often a symptom that accompanies anemia, subclinical hypoglycemia (low blood sugar), food allergies, etc. Hypothyroidism often manifests emotionally as depression. Depression commonly follows bouts of anger (liver disorder), and is a common problem with the elderly (often because of imbalanced diet). Most prevalent in the fifth through seventh decades of life, depression may also be a side-effect of oral contraceptives.

Self-test: When six or more of the following symptoms are present, this indicates severe depression and generally requires professional (medical, nutritional and/or psychotherapeutic) counseling:
1. Loss of appetite (or overeating)
2. Have considered suicide often
3. Crying frequently
4. Feeling lonely often
5. Have trouble focusing mentally
6. Feeling a sense of worthlessness
7. Difficulty with memory
8. Easily upset by small matters
9. Withdrawal from family, friends, associates
10. Regular sense of fatigue
11. Little or no interest in sex
12. Sleep problems (too much or insomnia)

Foot points: Adrenals; Liver; Gallbladder.

DERMATITIS: (also see: Acne; Impetigo, eczema; Skin; etc.): An inflammation of the skin. Dry or cracked skin is often a symptom of vitamin A or B complex deficiency.

Foot points: Lungs; Colon; Thyroid.

DIABETES (diabetes mellitus — also see: Pancreas; Spleen; etc.): A complex disease resulting from the underproduction of insulin, a vital chemical in the body's handling of sugar. (Note: Acupuncture, done professionally with needles, may be very helpful in controlling diabetes).

Foot points: Liver; Pancreas; Spleen; Adrenals; Kidneys; Thyroid; Stomach; Pituitary.

DIAPHRAGM: The muscular-tendonous partition that separates the chest (thorax) from the upper abdomen.

Foot points: Diaphragm.

DIARRHEA (loose, runny bowels — also see: DYSEN-TERY; "Traveler's diarrhea"; Gastrointestinal system; etc.): This condition may be symptomatic of any number of minor or major problems. If the condition continues for more than several days, dehydration may occur. It is primarily a disorder of the spleen and pancreas, in traditional Oriental theory. If this condition continues, get medical attention.

Foot points: Colon; Stomach; Spleen; Liver; Gall-bladder.

DIVERTICULITIS, DIVERTICULOSIS: See COLON; Constipation; GASTROINTESTINAL SYSTEM; etc.

Foot points: Kidneys.

DREAMING, EXCESSIVE (also see: INSOMNIA, etc.):
Frequent, sleep-disturbing mental activities which, in
traditional Oriental theory, are thought to be an
imbalance within the heart, small intestine,
pericardium ("heart protector") and endocrine system.

(Note: Dreaming may be an important indicator to the
state of health — even give advance warning about
impending health problems. If you suffer recurring,
frequent health-related dreams, see your doctor or
other health-care professional).

Foot points: Heart; Gallbladder.

DUODENUM: See Small intestine.

DYSENTERY (also see: Diarrhea; Gastrointestinal system;
etc.): An easily spread disease usually found in
tropical, overcrowded conditions. It originates in
contaminated food and/or water. There are several types
of dysentery, and their symptoms include severe
abdominal pain, frequent bowel movements (perhaps 25 or
30 per day — or more), loose-to-liquid stool, usually
flecked with blood, pus and/or mucus. Children are most
affected by this dangerous disease which is often
confused with cholera. And, like cholera, medical
attention is urgently required. (Note: Prolonged
bouts of amoebic dysentery may cause other problems
such as liver and/or lung abscesses, etc.).

Foot points: Colon; Stomach; Spleen.

DYSPEPSIA: See Flatulence; etc.

DYSPNEA (also see: RESPIRATORY SYSTEM; Asthma; etc.): Difficult or labored breathing usually symptomatic of an underlying disease or problem. It occurs when the capacity of the sufferer's breathing apparatus is temporarily unable to meet his body's demands, and often appears when breathing is reduced below 70% of maximum capacity. The sufferer may sense he is suffocating and thus panic, making the condition worse.

Since dyspnea is often a symptom of serious imbalance within the respiratory system, it is important to seek medical attention for this condition.

Foot points: (?) Lungs; Heart; Adrenals.

EAR (also see: Deafness, sudden, acute; HEARING DIFFICULTIES; Tinnitus; etc.): Includes the outer, middle and inner ear. A complete "micro-acupressure" healing system is found in the outer ear, making it a vital organ of health. The ear is considered to be a "product" of — and controlled by — the kidneys, according to traditional Oriental therapists.
Earaches, one of the most common ear disorders, often arise from bowel problems, such as constipation.

Foot points: Ear; Kidneys; Bladder (urinary); Eustachian tubes.

ECZEMA: See Impetigo and eczema.

EDEMA (dropsy): An excessive accumulation of fluid in the body's tissues. Generally, edema is a chronic problem. Since this condition often accompanies cardiovascular disorders, seek medical attention.

continued next page...

Foot points: Kidneys; Stomach; Liver; Pancreas; Spleen; affected bodily area.

ELBOW (including "tennis elbow" — also see: Arm; etc.):

Foot points: Elbow; Arm.

ENDOCRINE GLANDS (also see individual glands in this system): Various glands that secrete hormones directly into the bloodstream (vs. into another organ). Included in this system are the thyroid, parathyroid, thymus, pancreas, pituitary, adrenals, ovaries and testes (testicles). In certain traditional schools of thought (e.g., hatha yoga), this is the body's primary system by which other organs/functions are controlled. The glands within the system are highly interdependent, and the substances they synthesize — hormones — directly or indirectly control numerous bodily functions (e.g., growth, sexual development/function, metabolism, electrolyte balance, etc.). In short, hormones control the rate/intensity of numerous other biochemical or automatic functions and a dysfunction of one gland in the system necessarily means a dysfunction of several others. Any self-treatment of this system should be done only with caution and restraint.

Foot points: (?) Individual glands of the endocrine system (e.g., Adrenals, Thyroid, etc.).

EPIGLOTTIS (also see: Larynx; Throat; etc.): That elastic cartilage in the throat which protects the glottis while swallowing.

Foot points: Epiglottis.

EPILEPSY AND EPILEPTIC SEIZURES: A brain disorder
not clearly understood. There are a number of types of
epileptic attacks; the most dramatic is the grand mal
seizure. This may last from two to five minutes and
generally includes loss of consciousness, loss of
muscular control, rapid tensing and relaxing of the
muscles of the extremities, etc. No pressure-point
stimulation should be used during a seizure; instead,
try to help the sufferer avoid injuring himself,
especially his tongue. If possible, place a cloth-
wrapped stick between his teeth to prevent him from
biting his tongue.

The sufferer should not immediately get up and move
around, as this may trigger another seizure; instead he
should be made as comfortable as possible with his
clothing loosened. (Note: Onset of this dysfunction
usually occurs between ages three and fifteen years.)

Foot points: Bladder (urinary); Intestine, small;
Heart; Colon; Thyroid.

EUSTACHIAN TUBES (also see: Ear; Hearing difficulties;
Neck; Throat; etc.): The auditory tube.

Foot points: Eustachian tubes.

EYE (also see: Cataracts; Conjunctivitis): According to
traditional Oriental therapists, the eye is a product
or "child" of the liver — disorders of the eye
indicate an imbalance or malfunction in the liver (and
its companion organ, the gallbladder).

Foot points: Eye; Liver; Gallbladder; Stomach; Colon.

FACE (including facial neuralgia, etc. — also see: SKIN; Head; and specific areas, such as: Ear; Eye; Mouth; etc.):

Foot points: Forward (direction of toes) quarter of foot; all toes.

FATIGUE: Tiredness and lack of energy due to physical and/or mental exertion. Generally less serious than exhaustion, it is a substantial, though temporary, loss of strength.
    "Low energy" is one of the most common complaints from a person suffering from hypoglycemia, anemia, depression, "hidden" food allergies, etc. Since each of these may be a medical condition, if fatigue continues, seek professional attention.

Foot points: See ENDOCRINE GLANDS.

FEVER CONTROL CENTERS: Fever is that state of bodily temperature beyond the normal 98.6° F. or 37° C. It is a defense mechanism; the body produces an inhospitable climate for "intruders," foreign bodies, parasites, etc., in an effort to remove their threat or to "neutralize" them. It is a natural process and may be symptomatic of many problems.

(Note: Fever is a beneficial defensive and cleansing reaction — it is probably best to avoid trying to interfere with this vital process unless the fever is dangerously high.)

Foot points: Pituitary.

FINGERS: See Hand.

FITS: See Epilepsy and epileptic seizures; etc.

FLATULENCE (also see: Abdomen, lower; Gastrointestinal system; etc.): The presence of excessive gas in the stomach, intestines or anywhere in the gastrointestinal system. (Note: Flatulence arises from liver/gallbladder activity, in traditional Oriental theory. It is "normal" — that is, when consuming the average, Western diet — to expel gas ten to fifteen times daily; substantially more than that probably indicates at least a "hidden" food allergy and/or repressed, hostile emotions).

Foot points: Liver; Colon; Gallbladder.

FLU: See Colds and influenza.

FOOT (including ankle, toes, etc.):

Foot points: Ankle; Foot, feet.

FRACTURES (broken bone — also see Bones; specific area where the fracture has occurred such as Arm, etc.): A broken or splintered bone. Acupressure techniques do not replace standard Western first-aid or emergency measures such as splints, casts, or other immobilizing wrappings and coverings.

Foot points: Use corresponding affected area.

FRIGIDITY (sexual — also see SEXUAL DRIVE; Sexual organs, etc.): Sexual unresponsiveness within a female partner. (Note: A much more in-depth program for healing sexual disorders is found in this author's book, "HOW TO ENJOY SEX MORE WITH ACUGENICS").

Foot points: Kidneys; Lungs; Heart; Spleen.

FROSTBITE (including: Chilblain; Immersion Foot; Pernio; and Trench Foot — also see: Skin; and specific areas affected, etc.): The result of prolonged exposure to damp or dry cold. The most severe condition is frostbite, where the tissue of the affected part of the body is destroyed by freezing. Blood circulation is stopped to the affected area; unless rapidly treated, this will become gangrenous and amputation may be required.

Currently there is general agreement among authorities that immediate thawing in warm water as soon as the threat of refreezing passes is the best choice. But it will be painful. Never rub a frostbitten area, even with snow. Get medical help immediately.

Foot points: Lungs; plus corresponding bodily area points.

GALLBLADDER (also see: Flatulence; etc.): A hollow
organ located near the liver, in the upper right-hand
quarter of the abdomen area, beneath or behind the
ribcage. Its function is the accumulation and storage
of mucus and bile. Pain or discomfort in that part of
the upper abdomen, especially after eating, could
indicate gallbladder or liver problems.

In traditional Oriental theory, the gallbladder is
one of the primary twelve organs and is mated with the
liver, the organ from which it "blooms" during fetal
development. As such, its emotional "chores" are
anger, decision-making, depression, etc. Symptoms
of disorder and imbalance within this organ include
flatulence; pain or colic in the upper, right quadrant
of the abdomen; nausea; bowel distress; difficulty in
making decisions for oneself; and, of course,
gallstones. (Note: About half of all gallbladder
"attacks" occur from April through May; in traditional
Oriental theory, this corresponds to the time — spring
— when the gallbladder and liver organ "team" are most
active.) (For more in-depth techniques for healing
this organ, see this author's THE NATURAL HEALER'S
ACUPRESSURE HANDBOOK, VOLUME II.)

Foot points: Liver; Gallbladder.

GALLSTONES (also see: GALLBLADDER): Crystallized
bits of bile, composed primarily of cholesterol. This
condition — which afflicts females far more often than
males — is so common (esp. in older people) that as
many as one person in five suffers from gallstones by
age 65. (Note: Cancer of the gallbladder is nearly
always preceded by gallstones.) The period of
pregnancy is also a typical time for gallstones to
form.

continued next page...

While the existence of gallstones may be symptom-free until they actually pass, common symptoms include cramping pain (which has been compared to childbirth), bloating, belching, food intolerance, bad breath, etc. Gallstones may mimic brain tumors, appendicitis, pancreatitis, ulcers, etc.

Foot points: Liver; Gallbladder; Pancreas.

GASTRITIS (acid indigestion — also see: STOMACH; Flatulence; Gastrointestinal system; etc.): Inflammation of the stomach, usually due to acid/alkaline imbalance. Symptoms of too much or too little stomach acid (HCL) may be similar.

Foot points: Stomach; Liver; Spleen; Pancreas.

GASTROINTESTINAL SYSTEM (also see: Abdomen, lower and upper; Flatulence; Stomach; etc.): The stomach and intestinal portions of the digestive tract.

Foot points: Stomach; Liver; Gallbladder; Intestine, small; Colon; Spleen; Pancreas.

GENITAL WEAKNESS, PAIN and/or DYSFUNCTION: See Gonorrhea; Sexual organs; etc.

GENITOURINARY SYSTEM (also see: Kidneys; Bladder, urinary; Cystitis; Urinary control centers; SEXUAL DRIVE; Sexual organs; etc.): The system whose job is the excretion of urine; it includes the kidneys, urinary bladder, ureters and urethra, as well as the internal and external organs of reproduction (sex organs). (Note: In good health, urine should be slightly acidic — with a pH of about 5.5 — especially upon the morning's first urination.)

Foot points: Kidneys; Bladder (urinary); Ureter tubes; Sex organs; Adrenals.

GINGIVITIS (bleeding gums, unhealthy gums — also see: MOUTH; TOOTH, TEETH; Toothache; etc.): A condition which may be disease-linked, although more often it arises from improper and irregular care of the gums and teeth.

Foot points: (?) Colon; Lungs; Tooth, teeth.

GLANDS, SWOLLEN: See LYMPH GLANDS.

GLAUCOMA (also see: EYE; etc.): A group of disorders of the eye, characterized by abnormal elevation of intraocular pressure, hardening of the eyeball, restricted field of vision, halos seen around artificial lights and a general loss of visual power. If glaucoma is suspected — or there is a family history of this disorder — get a complete physical eye examination (not just a tonometric pressure reading, since this can be misleading).

Foot points: (?) Eye; Liver.

GONORRHEA (also see: Sexual organs; etc.): A venereal
disease primarily involving the mucous membranes of the
genitourinary tract and/or rectum. Sometimes the eye
is involved, as well. Its symptoms include painful
urination, pus seepage from the urinary tract, and
various genitourinary infections Gonorrhea is primarily
spread by sexual intercourse. Get medical help
immediately both for treatment and to help stop the
spread of this disease.

Foot points: (?) Sex organs.

GOUT (also see: Arthritis): A recurrent attack of acute
arthritis that mostly strikes the big toe. The main
symptom is mild-to-excruciating pain in or about the
big toe. Sometimes crystal formations are found along
the edges of the ear. Gout is caused by the improper
metabolism of uric acid and may be triggered by an
excess of wine or various rich foods.

Foot points: Affected bodily area.

HAIR (esp. graying — also see: Baldness; Dandruff;
etc.): Hair (on the head) is thought to be a product of
— and thus controlled by — the kidneys (and/or
lungs), by traditional Oriental therapists. As such, it
is part of the excretory system.

Foot points: Thyroid (use cautiously).

HAND (including fingers — also see: Arm; Wrist; etc):

Foot points: Arm; Shoulder; Elbow.

-47-

HANGOVER (also see: Flatulence; Intoxication; etc.):
The disagreeable aftereffects from drug or alcohol
abuse. Its symptoms often include nausea, headache,
indigestion, diarrhea, etc. If this condition occurs
after taking only a small amount of the intoxicant, it
generally indicates an allergy to the intoxicant or one
of its ingredients.

Foot points: (?) Stomach; Liver.

HAY FEVER (also see: Allergies, non-specific; Eye;
Nasal congestion; etc.): Common name for allergic
rhinitis. Hay fever is a catchall term to describe a
loosely knit group of allergic reactions triggered by
pollination of various plants or weeds.

Foot points: Nose; Sinuses; Lungs.

HEAD (also see: Ear; Eye; Face; Headache; Mouth; Neck;
Whiplash; etc.): Any injury to the head is potentially
dangerous. Signs of shock should be carefully watched
for as well as signs of concussion. Fracture of the
skull should be suspected, especially if there are
differences between the size of the pupils, or bleeding
from the nose, ears and/or mouth. Keep the victim
quiet and get medical help immediately.

Foot points: (?) Brain; Pineal; Pituitary.

HEADACHES (also see: Head; Migraine; Pain control centers; etc.): May be symptomatic of many problems and diseases. If headache persists, or is a frequent problem, get medical help. The following headaches which require prompt professional attention are those that strike without apparent cause; awaken you from a deep sleep; are accompanied by confusion or convulsions; change character after having a long history of sameness; are constant, daily or frequent; are localized in a specific place (e.g., in ear, eye, etc.); follow a blow to the head; are recurrent in children.

"Common" headaches (there are more than 60 kinds of headache) are usually a symptom of imbalance within the digestive organs, and are frequently triggered by stress and tension.

Foot points: Liver; Spleen; Stomach; Gallbladder; Colon; Adrenals.

HEARING DIFFICULTIES (also see: Deafness; Ear; etc.): Hearing is associated with the kidneys, in traditional Oriental theory. There are three major kinds of hearing loss: Nerve loss (aging, following fever, etc.); conductive loss (build-up of earwax, etc.); functional loss (often psychological). Hearing difficulties may also forewarn of heart and/or kidney disorders (esp. inner ear disorders).

Foot points: Ear; Kidneys; Bladder (urinary) Eustachian tubes.

HEART (also see: Angina pectoris; Chest; Heart attack, heart failure; etc.): One of the twelve primary organs in traditional Oriental theory, the heart — and its companion organ, the small intestine — are primarily responsible for blood (and energy) circulation. It is considered the "king" of organs and the most vulnerable — thus, except when no alternatives exist, self-treatment of any known heart conditions should be avoided.

Early warning signs of potential heart failure include edema (esp. of the ankles); breathlessness following mild exercise (e.g., after climbing stairs); a hacking-type cough that immediately ceases when one stands up but comes on when lying down or sitting); enlarged fingertips and/or nose; frequent urination at night; tiny lumps, nodules or blood spots under skin; raised orange spots under the skin, especially around the wrist; double-jointed wrists and fingers, accompanied by skin and hands that bruise easily; long, thin spider-like fingers that seem to be double-jointed; aggressive, time-urgent and competitive behavior, among others. (Note: Unusual depression and/or fatigue — as well as a reduced sexual drive and numerous other "unrelated" symptoms — may also be early warning indicators of heart disease, attack, etc. For more in-depth techniques for healing this organ, see this author's THE NATURAL HEALER'S ACUPRESSURE HANDBOOK, VOLUME II.)

Foot points: Heart; Intestine, small; Bladder (urinary).

HEART ATTACK, HEART FAILURE (also see: Angina pectoris; Chest; Heart; Pain control centers; etc.): A major disturbance of the heart caused by either blockage of a coronary artery (heart attack) or inadequate pumping of the heart (heart failure). Symptoms of heart attack include severe pain or crushing pressure beneath the breastbone (sternum), a feeling of apprehension, shortness of breath, profuse sweating, and nausea and/or vomiting. The pain may first appear on the left side of the upper body before moving into the chest.

Symptoms of heart failure include edema (swelling of hands and feet), bluish-purple coloring of the skin, lips, fingernails, ears, etc., chest pains, anxiety and shortness of breath, especially when lying down.

Get medical help immediately, and do not consume food or water when any heart disturbance is suspected.

Emergency tactics: A) If heart attack occurs, force yourself to cough constantly until you can reach help; since there are only about 10-20 seconds before losing consciousness, begin coughing immediately (forced coughing simulates cardiopulmonary resuscitation or CPR).
B) Bite the tips of fifth (little) fingers (inside and outside, not top and bottom — this triggers two vital acupressure points).

Foot points: (?) Heart.

HEEL (also see: Foot; etc.): Chronic heel problems may be an early warning indicator of heart problems.

Foot points: Foot, feet.

HEMORRHAGE (bleeding — also see: Menstrual difficulties; Nosebleed; and specific affected body areas): Blood flows through vessels such as veins and arteries, carrying oxygen and food to the cells and carrying away waste. If something happens to rupture the vessels, blood escapes; or disease may allow the blood to escape through unruptured vessels (diapedisis). Both are considered as hemorrhage; if enough blood escapes, death occurs.

Foot points: Corresponding bodily area.

HEMORRHOIDS (piles — also see: Anus; Pain control centers; Rectum; etc.): An enlarged, expanded vein in the lower rectal and/or anal wall. Complications may include inflammation, bleeding, pain and/or itching and possibly clotting (thrombosis). Permanently curing hemorrhoids usually means a change in diet, toilet habits and/or mental attitudes.

Hemorrhoids — which are common during pregnancy — are caused by excess pressure on the rectum (usually from constipation or unassimilated foods). They are often accompanied by gum problems and disorders. Hemorrhoids which bleed are common, but regular bleeding from anus requires medical attention.

Foot points: Anus; Sigmoid colon; Rectum; Prostate; Spleen.

HEPATITIS: See JAUNDICE; LIVER. This is an inflammation of the liver which is dangerous and may be communicable. Get medical help immediately. (Note: If skin has yellow pallor or cast, see JAUNDICE.)

Foot points: (?) Liver; Bladder (urinary); Gallbladder.

HERNIA (rupture — also see: Abdomen, lower etc.): An abnormal protrusion of the intestine through the abdominal muscle wall or cavity. Hernia is often caused by lifting an excessive weight or improperly hoisting a load. Ordinarily, a small-to-large bulge will appear somewhere upon the abdomen; and there may be some pain. The ultimate danger lies in the possibility of cutting off the source of blood to the protruding bowel.

Foot points: Corresponding bodily points.

HERPES SIMPLEX VIRUS II (genital herpes — also see Shingles; etc.): A highly contagious viral infection primarily of the genital and/or anal areas. (Note: Techniques should be started at the first hint of an impending outbreak.)

Foot points: (?) Affected bodily points.

HERPES ZOSTER VIRUS: See SHINGLES.

HICCOUGH (hiccup) CONTROL CENTER: With older persons, especially, hiccoughs are often associated with hardening of the arteries (arteriosclerosis). Generally caused by a spasmodic contraction of the diaphragm due to irritation of the phrenic nerve.

Foot points: Diaphragm (?).

HIGH BLOOD PRESSURE: See Hypertension.

HIP (also see: Buttocks; etc.):

Foot points: Hip.

HIVES AND RASH (urticaria — also see: Allergies, non-specific; Skin; etc.): Sudden or rapid appearance of intensive, itching welts on the skin. They may appear in crops over wide areas of the body, tend to last a day or so, and are generally associated with allergic reactions.

In severe cases, hives may affect the mucous membrane areas; edema may constrict the vocal area (glottis), creating possibly fatal distress. Get medical help immediately.

Foot points: Use corresponding bodily area points.

HOARSENESS (also see: Laryngitis; Throat; etc.): Irritated or phlegm-coated throat and vocal area, causing raspy or strained voice. Chronic hoarseness should have medical attention.

Foot points: (?) Lungs; Bronchial tubes; Larynx; Throat; Trachea; Tonsils.

HUNGER CONTROL CENTERS: To temporarily ease hunger. For further information and techniques, see this author's HOW TO LOSE WEIGHT EASILY WITH ACU-GENICS.

Foot points: (?) Stomach; Liver; Gallbladder.

HYPERACTIVITY: A state of restlessness and frequent movement, especially found in children.

Foot points: See HYPOGLYCEMIA, NERVOUSNESS, etc.

HYPERTENSION (high blood pressure): Its symptoms are as vague as the origin of the disease. Besides increased blood pressure, there may be dizziness, fatigue, insomnia, palpitations, weakness and head-aches, etc. Hypertension occurs from the stricture of blood vessels, caused either by fats (and other "mechanical" processes) or through fear or other psychophysical means, but the result is similar — blood is forced through too small an opening.
     Untreated hypertension is dangerous — take steps immediately and get professional advice. Nearly always, high blood pressure is at least partially food-related — important changes in diet are essential; and if taken, such steps are often enough to control hypertension without drugs or medications (see this author's A WAY OF EATING FOR PLEASURE AND HEALTH).

Foot points: (?) Kidneys; Adrenals; Colon (all).

HYPOGLYCEMIA (low blood sugar — also see: Diabetes mellitus; Spleen; Pancreas; FATIGUE; etc.): A condition about which little is known, but is thought by some nutrition authorities to affect millions. The problem is too much insulin and/or not enough "blood sugar," which may trigger insulin shock in severe cases. Its symptoms may be similar to diabetes mellitus, a problem with which it is often confused.

continued next page...

While "hypoglycemia" means "low blood sugar," in its pre-clinical, common form, it is coming to mean an umbrella syndrome that includes numerous symptoms (e.g., anger, fatigue, etc.) that are primarily triggered by an allergy to sugar or sugary foods and drinks.

Hypoglycemia typically occurs about two/three hours following a meal (sooner — usually within a half-hour — following sugary foods, smoking, taking alcoholic and/or caffeinated drinks, etc.). Its symptoms include: Flushing; pallid/sallow skin; feeling of faintness; hyperactivity (esp. in children); IRRITABILITY; low emotional control; chills; HUNGER; trembling; headaches; dizziness; weakness; convulsions; etc.

Foot points: (?) Liver; Pancreas; Spleen; Adrenals; Heart; Kidneys; Bladder (urinary); Pituitary; Brain; Gallbladder; Intestine, small.

ILEO-CECUM (also see: Colon; Gastrointestinal system; Small intestine; etc.): The "doorway" between the small intestine and the colon, found in the lower right quadrant of the abdomen. In Oriental literature, it is said to be "controlled" by the kidneys.

Foot points: Ileo-cecum.

IMPETIGO and ECZEMA (also see: Skin, etc.): Skin disorders whose symptoms are crusty, yellowish formations and pustules (impetigo) or drier, more reddened lesions (eczema); or they may look similar.

Foot points: (?) Adrenals; Kidneys; Lungs; plus corresponding body area points.

IMPOTENCE (Sexual — also see: SEXUAL DRIVE; Sexual organs; etc.): Inability in a male to have complete sexual intercourse. It is common for most males to suffer this condition occasionally. But when this mostly psychological condition (primarily an affliction of the kidneys, in traditional Oriental theory) occurs more than 25% of the time, it probably indicates severe, nutritional imbalance (or maybe a side-effect of present medication, alcoholism, drug abuse, etc.). At that point, professional help is suggested, especially since frequent impotence may also be a symptom of an underlying organic disease or disorder (e.g., diabetes).

The healthy male should be able to have a satisfying sex life for his entire life. Impotence generally results from insufficient blood to the penis, malfunctioning nervous system or abnormal amounts of male hormones.

In a healthy male, sexual desire is strongest in cool or cold weather and is lowest in hot weather, when frequent sexual orgasms tend to damage the kidneys and heart.

More complete information on this subject is found in this author's HOW TO ENJOY SEX MORE WITH ACUGENICS.

Foot points: Liver; Pancreas; Spleen; Heart; Kidneys; Bladder (urinary); Sex organs; Prostate.

INFECTION: The "invasion" of the body by various organisms such as hostile bacteria or viruses.

Foot points: Use corresponding bodily area points.

INFLAMMATIONS (also see: Arthritis, minor; Sores; affected bodily areas; etc.): The reaction of tissue to injury, etc., characterized by soreness, heat, swelling, etc.

Foot points: Use corresponding bodily area points.

INFLUENZA: See COLDS and INFLUENZA.

INSOMNIA: Sleeplessness and mild restlessness; prolonged difficulty in getting to sleep.

Foot points: Liver; Gallbladder; Kidneys; Bladder (urinary); Pancreas; Spleen.

INTESTINAL PROBLEMS: See Constipation (costiveness); Diarrhea; Dysentery; Gastrointestinal System; Flatulence; Pain control centers; etc.

INTOXICATION (also see: Hangover; etc.): Mild or severe poisioning from the abuse of alcohol, medication, or drugs.

(NOTE: THE FOLLOWING ACUPRESSURE TECHNIQUES ARE FOR EMERGENCY USE ONLY — INTOXICATION IS ONE OF THE CONTRAINDICATED CONDITIONS FOR ACUPRESSURE.)

Foot points: (?) Liver; Spleen; Lungs; Pancreas.

ITCHING; ITCHY SKIN (also see: SKIN; Impetigo and eczema; etc.): Frequent itching may be an early warning of kidney disorder, diabetes mellitus, gout, thyroid dysfunction or even leukemia, cancer (carcinoma) or Hodgkin's Disease. If itching continues or increases, seek medical attention and diagnosis. (Note: Itchy skin — esp. if repeatedly in a specific area — may be the system's "shout" for acupunture upon that point; itching at various acupoints about the skin is the body-mind's own way of doing acupuncture therapy upon itself.)

Foot points: (?) Liver; Bladder (urinary); Gall-bladder; Spleen; Stomach; Colon (all).

JAUNDICE (also see: Liver; etc.): Yellowing of the skin or mucous membranes, and secretions with bile pigment. Jaundice may occur from a number of causes, but is generally disease-linked. The liver is primarily or secondarily affected; this is the bile-producing organ. Jaundice that appears suddenly — or suddenly deepens — may indicate passage and lodging of a gallstone in the common bile duct, causing the bile to become blocked, thus yellowing the skin. (Note: Jaundice is very common in newborn infants — some doctors feel that an allergy to breast milk may be involved.)

Foot points: (?) Adrenals; Kidneys; Liver; Lungs.

JAW, LOWER (also see: Dental work; Jaw, upper; Mouth; Toothache; etc.): Jaw pain, difficulty in chewing, may indicate vitamin B complex deficiency.

Foot points: Tongue; Tooth, teeth.

JAW, UPPER (also see: Dental work; Jaw, lower; Mouth; Toothache; etc.):

Foot points: Tongue; Tooth, teeth.

KIDNEYS (also see: Back, lower and/or upper; Bladder, urinary; GENITOURINARY SYSTEM; KIDNEY STONES; NEPHRITIS; etc.): The pair of primary organs, located in the body at the level of the elbows, which are the "parents" of the genitourinary system. In traditional Oriental theory, the kidneys — and their companion organ, the urinary bladder — are responsible for "producing" the responses to fear, sexual hunger, etc. They are also said to control hearing and hair (on the head). (For more in-depth techniques for healing this organ, see this author's THE NATURAL HEALER'S ACUPRESSURE HANDBOOK, VOLUME II.)

Foot points: Kidneys; Adrenals; Bladder (urinary).

KIDNEY STONES: See GENITOURINARY SYSTEM; Kidneys; STONES, KIDNEY OR BLADDER; etc.

KNEE (also see: Foot; Leg; Thigh; etc.):

Foot points: Knee.

LARYNGITIS (also see: Bronchitis; Colds and influenza; Hoarseness; Larynx; Respiratory system; Throat; etc.): An inflammation of the larynx or voice box which causes a hoarseness or inability to vocalize sound. Chronic or acute, it may be caused by a number of factors.

continued next page...

<u>Foot points</u>: Larynx; Lungs; Throat.

LARYNX (also see: Laryngitis; Pharnyx; RESPIRATORY
SYSTEM; Throat; etc.): The "voice box," found between
the tongue and the trachea. It is part of the
respiratory system and is controlled by the lungs.

<u>Foot points</u>: Larynx; Lungs; Throat.

LEG (also see: Foot; Knee; Thigh: etc. — for leg
cramps, see CRAMPS and SPASMS, MUSCULAR):

<u>Foot points</u>: Foot, feet; Knee; Hip.

LEG CRAMPS (at night): See CRAMPS and SPASMS,
MUSCULAR.

LIVER (also see: Gallbladder; Jaundice; Pancreas;
Spleen; etc.): The largest gland or secreting organ in
the body. Its functions are not totally understood,
but it plays a major role in the digestive process.
Symptoms of a liver disorder may include pain and/or
discomfort behind the bottom of the rib cage and are
sometimes confused with problems of the gallbladder.
    In traditional Oriental theory, the liver produces
— or is "responsible" for — the eyes, muscles, moving
the bowels, flatulence, aggressive drive, anger,
depression, etc. It is a primary organ for vitality and
physical force or strength.

continued next page...

The liver — and its companion, the gallbladder —
also produce digestive enzymes and act as a filter
between the heart and intestine, producing red blood
cells and processing waste nitrogen into urea. The
liver is the body's fastest "self-regenerator" organ.
(For more in-depth techniques for healing this organ,
see this author's THE NATURAL HEALER'S ACUPRES-
SURE HANDBOOK, VOLUME II.)

Foot points: Liver; Gallbladder; Pancreas; Spleen;
Bladder (urinary).

LOCKJAW: See Tetanus.

LOW BLOOD SUGAR: See Hypoglycemia.

LUMBAGO (also see: Back, lower and/or upper; Pain
control centers; Sciatica; etc.): Aching in the lower
to middle back region.

Foot points: See BACK.

LUNGS (also see: Asthma; Bronchitis; Colon; Cough; Chest; Respiratory System; etc.): Primary organs for handling air and which, in traditional Oriental theory, are coupled with the colon (large intestine). They "control" the nose and breathing passages, the sense of smell, the skin (and bodily — not scalp — hair); the emotions they produce/store are thought to be, in part, grief, anxiety, resentment and sorrow. The lungs play a critical part in the regulation of bodily temperature (via perspiration) and the elimination of fluids from the body. They are also the "home" of animal drive, sense of reason and wisdom, the sense of survival and the will to live. (For more in-depth techniques for healing this organ, see this author's THE NATURAL HEALER'S ACUPRESSURE HANDBOOK, VOLUME II.)

Foot points: Bronchial tubes; Lungs.

LYMPH GLANDS or NODES (also see: SPLEEN; etc.): The system for carrying lymph (a bodily fluid) that involves the following glands: Pineal; pituitary; adrenals; thymus; thyroid; tonsils; appendix; adenoids; and various other nodes. Its primary chore is cleansing blood of impurities. In traditional Oriental Theory, the "Triple Warmer" (a body-regulation function that has no Western counterpart) is said to control the lymph system, while the spleen (including the pancreas) and its companion organ, the stomach, are said to be the "parents" of this system. (NOTE: All following acupressure points to be used with restraint and caution.)

Foot points: Adrenals; Appendix; Lymph nodes (drainage); Pancreas; Pineal; Pituitary; Spleen; Stomach; Thymus; Thyroid; Tonsils.

MASTITIS (also see: BREASTS; etc.): An inflammation of the breast, in which breast becomes swollen, reddened, knotty and/or tender to the touch. It is frequent among nursing mothers.

Foot points: (?) Breasts; Stomach.

MASTOID PROCESS: (also see: Ear; etc.): The breast or nipple-shaped bone of the skull, just behind the ear.

Foot points: (?) Ear.

MENOPAUSE (also see: MENSTRUAL DIFFICULTIES; etc.): The so-called "change of life" experienced by females in middle age, considered to have occurred when a female stops her period for over a year. Those who begin menstruation early are characteristically the last to undergo menopause.

The most noticeable symptom is a gradual-to-sudden cessation of menstruation. Other symptoms of this condition may include "hot flashes," itching skin, constipation, heart palpitations, headache, dizziness, emotional changes, etc. (Note: Males also undergo menopause, which is chiefly characterized by shrinkage of sex organs and the emotional discomfort which that may bring). Discontinuance of the production of hormones (estrogen and progesterone) and menopause are linked intimately together. Endocrine changes in younger women can cause hormonal disruption, bringing on early menopause.

continued next page...

(Note: Menopause is not an absolute time clock
process, though it is extremely common — there are
reports of 70-and 80-year-old females giving birth to
healthy babies. Acupressure techniques may delay/ease
the onset/difficulty of menopause, being especially
helpful in the continued production of female
hormones.)

Foot points: (?) Sex organs; Pituitary; Brain.

MENSTRUAL DIFFICULTIES: (including Dysmenorrhea,
Menorrhagia, Leukorrhea, etc. — also see: Ovaries;
Abdomen, lower; Pain control centers; Sexual organs;
etc.): Female reproductive organs generally function
well for about 30 years after onset of menstruation
(monthly fertility cycle). Slight variations in cycle
or accompanying symptoms are not significant; but
sudden and/or major changes — such as complete
cessation of menstruation even when not pregnant —
require immediate medical attention (esp. non-menstrual
vaginal bleeding).
    Menstrual difficulties may include: Menorrhagia
(loss of large amounts of blood); dysmenorrhea (painful
menstruation); amenorrhea (absence of menstrual
period); leukorrhea or the "whites" (non-bloody vaginal
discharge); etc.

Foot points: Thyroid; Spleen; Stomach; Kidneys;
Bladder (urinary); Liver.

MIGRAINE (also see: Headache; etc.): A particularly severe headache, often said to be associated with a malfunctioning liver by Oriental doctor-philosophers. It is characterized by periodic, rapid onsets that often center in or around one or both eyes and may be accompanied by other painful, unpleasant symptoms. Vomiting, nausea, loss of appetite and strength are not uncommon.

True migraine — often called "sick headache" — differs from the many other kinds of headaches (some doctors claim there are more than 60 types of headaches) in that it usually occurs on one side of the head and follows a rather consistent pattern. Disturbance in vision is also a common symptom for this tension-related headache.

The "migraine personality" is one that is tense, rigid, hard-driving, conscientious and always striving for perfection. Psychotherapy — with the goal of loosening, easing and relaxing these personality aspects — may be most helpful.

Nearly 75% of all migraines are suffered by females, especially near their menstrual periods. Migraine is often hereditary and is thought to affect about 5% of the population.

Foot points: (?) Liver; Lungs.

MOUTH (also see: Dental work; Face; Gingivitis; Head; Jaw, lower; Jaw, upper; Palate, Parotid gland; Tongue; Toothache; etc.): The mouth is one of the body's most vulnerable areas to disturbances in nutrition, the endocrine system and in the process of metabolism.

continued next page...

Common symptoms of mouth disorders include: Canker sores; cold sores (herpes facialis); thrush (mouth ulcers); cracking at corners of mouth (cheilosis); chapped lips; foul and sticky mouth and tongue (usually indicates a liver imbalance); etc.

Foot points: Palate; Stomach; Spleen; Pancreas; Liver.

MULTIPLE SCLEROSIS (also see: Nerves; etc.): A disease of the central nervous system that primarily affects the white matter of the brain and spinal cord. It is a progressively degenerative disorder that tends to occur in "bouts" (some of which are triggered by high fever, injuries, pregnancy, etc.). Some of its many symptoms include blurred/double vision; speech difficulties; weakness in limbs; loss of bladder/bowel control; loss of balance; difficulty in walking; etc.

The disease tends to recur frequently with decreasing spans of "relief time" between bouts. While depression occurs, many M.S. patients exude a surprising sense of cheerfulness and optimism.

Foot points: Brain; Kidneys; Stomach; Spleen; Pancreas; Liver; Gallbladder.

MUMPS: An acute, painful and contagious viral disease. Its symptoms are generally an enlargement of one or both salivary glands — especially the parotid gland (located in front of and below the ear) — but may include attacks on other tissues such as the testicles, pancreas, etc.

continued next page...

Mumps is more dangerous to adults — especially adult males — than to children. It occurs mostly in the winter and spring months. Usually, a case of childhood mumps gives lifelong protection, and nearly a third of the people who contract this disease never realize they've had it.

Symptoms of mumps include: Pain under the ear (preceded by chills, fever, loss of appetite and/or headache, etc.); swelling of the parotid gland; puffiness on (usually only) one side of the face; difficulty in swallowing; etc. This usually lasts for a week to 10 days.

Foot points: (?) Adrenals; Lymph nodes; Neck; Throat; Palate.

MUSCLES (also see: Cramps and spasms, muscular; Sprains, muscular; Strains, muscular; etc.): Muscles are sub-organs of the body which, in traditional Oriental theory, are "children" of the liver and gallbladder; to a certain extent, they are also controlled by the spleen, pancreas and stomach.

Foot points: See specific areas; Liver; Gallbladder; Spleen; Pancreas; Stomach.

NASAL CONGESTION (catarrh — also see: Colds and influenza; Hay fever; Nose; Sinusitis; etc.): An inflammation of the nasal passages' mucous membranes combined with a mucus discharge.

Foot points: Lungs; Nose; Sinuses; Colon; Stomach.

NECK (also see: Whiplash; etc.):

Foot points: Neck.

NEPHRITIS (acute — also see: Genitourinary system; Kidneys, etc.): Inflammation of the kidneys. When chronic, it is called "Bright's Disease." It is usually characterized by: Fatigue; reduced sexual drive; lowered vitality; albumin in the urine; swelling in various parts of the body; etc. Nausea, vomiting and enlargement of the abdomen are also common.

Foot points: Kidneys; Adrenals.

NERVES (nervous system — also see Brain; NERV-OUSNESS; etc.): The control system for all muscular movements, including the brain, central and peripheral nervous system and spinal cord. Primary damage to the nervous system arises usually from poor nutrition and/or dysfunction of the endocrine glands.

Diseases of the nervous system include — but are not limited to — Parkinson's disease; multiple sclerosis; myasthenia gravis; neuralgia; neuritis; epilepsy; muscular dystrophy; Tay-Sach's disease; rheumatoid arthritis; etc.

Foot points: Brain; Nerves; Stomach; Kidneys; Bladder (urinary); Adrenals.

NERVOUSNESS (also see: Nerves; etc.): A state of mental and/or physical disarray, characterized by a lack of mental poise and composure, restlessness, impulsive and/or irrational behavior, purposeless activity, etc.

Nervousness is a catchall word that often refers to symptoms that have little to do with the nervous system, but are actually low-level fear reactions (kidney-urinary bladder imbalance).

Foot points: (?) Stomach; Kidneys; Bladder (urinary).

NEURALGIA (also see: Pain control centers; Trigeminal Neuralgia; specific areas affected, such as Arm; Hand; etc.): Aching sensitivity or brief, stabbing pains along the course of a nerve.

Foot points: Corresponding bodily area point(s).

NEURASTHENIA (neurasthenic neurosis — also see: NERVES; etc.): A group of symptoms which are generally related to nervous exhaustion (e.g., "low energy," weakness, various aches and pains, etc.).

Foot points: See NERVES.

NIGHTMARES (especially affecting children — also see: Nervousness; etc.): Frightening dreams. Primarily a disorder of childhood that passes by age six or seven. Frequent nightmares may indicate need for professional — esp. dietary — counseling.

Foot points: See DREAMING, EXCESSIVE.

NOSE (also see: Nasal congestion; Nosebleed; etc.): The external orifice of the respiratory system. In the traditional Oriental view, the nostrils and nasal passages are controlled by the lungs, while the external part is related to the heart.

Foot points: Nose.

NOSEBLEED (epistaxis — also see: Nose; etc.): A nasal hemorrhage which may be minor and simple or linked to more serious problems such as concussion. Any nosebleed that lasts more than ten or fifteen minutes requires immediate medical attention (since it usually indicates a more serious, underlying condition).

Foot points: Nose (?).

NUMBNESS: Local or general insensitivity (anesthesia) often coupled with sluggishness, "pins and needles" feeling, tingling, etc. Sudden or unexplained numbness calls for immediate medical attention, since it is usually a symptom of an underlying disorder.

Foot points: (?) Corresponding bodily area point(s).

OCCIPUT (back of head — also see: Head; Headache; Neck; etc.):

Foot points: Head; Neck.

OVARIES (also see: Menstrual difficulties; Sexual organs; etc.): The two female sex glands that germinate egg cells and provide internal secretions (hormones).

Most common ovarian problems are infections, cysts, tumors and stretching (or straining). When ovarian symptoms occur on the right side, they are easily mistaken for appendicitis. Gonorrhea (as well as tuberculosis) may be particularly harmful to fertility — as well as being a common cause of subsequent arthritis — so any infection of the ovaries or genitourinary system should have prompt, medical attention.

Foot points: Ovary; Adrenals.

PAIN CONTROL CENTERS (also see: Headache; Neuralgia; specific portions of body affected, such as Arm; Hand; etc.): Pain is one of the body's first lines of communication and defense and may arise from conditions in parts of the body away from the pain site. For chronic recurring pain, get medical help.

Foot points: Use corresponding bodily area points.

PALATE (also see: MOUTH; etc.): The roof of the mouth, composed of the "hard" and "soft" palates.

Foot points: Stomach; Spleen; Pancreas; Palate.

PANCREAS (also see: Diabetes; ENDOCRINE GLANDS; Hypoglycemia; SPLEEN; etc.): Located immediately beside the spleen (just behind the bottom of the ribcage and upper abdomen), this gland is responsible for the production of insulin, pancreatic juice, etc. It is a vital organ and is linked, in traditional Oriental theory, to both the spleen and the stomach. It is a prime organ in hypoglycemia (low blood sugar), and problems such as jaundice, diabetes mellitus or pancreatitis may develop from its malfunction. Deep, severe pain between the shoulder blades — especially in middle-aged-to-elderly males — calls for immediate medical attention, since that is a common symptom of pancreatic cancer. (Note: Pancreatitis, on the other hand — an inflammation of the pancreas — affects females more frequently than males. For more in-depth techniques for healing this organ, see this author's THE NATURAL HEALER'S ACUPRESSURE HANDBOOK, VOLUME II.)

Foot points: Spleen; Pancreas; Stomach.

PARALYSIS (also see: Numbness; etc.): Loss of sensation and muscle function due to injury to the nervous system and/or disease-linked destruction of the nervous connections. Partial or complete paralysis may even be triggered by psychological problems and conditions such as hysteria. Paralysis may affect specific areas of half the body (hemiplegia) or more. Get medical help immediately.

continued next page...

(Note: Paralysis due to brain damage is generally of the stiff or spastic type, whereas spinal disorders generally cause paralysis of the flaccid sort.)

Foot points: Use corresponding bodily area points.

PARASITES, INTERNAL (e.g., pinworms, hookworms, etc.): Symptoms (esp. of worms) often include: Restlessness (esp. at night); nose picking; teeth-grinding or gritting (during sleep); dry cough; anal itching (esp. at night); changes in bowel habits; weight loss or inability to gain weight (esp. tapeworms); etc. Internal parasites are extremely common, especially in those who keep dogs, cats and other affectionate pets. Numerous allergies or similar problems are parasite-"inspired" (e.g., a common form of asthma appears to arise as a weakened state produced by roundworms, transmitted by dogs).

Foot points: Use GASTROINTESTINAL points.

PARATHYROID GLANDS: See THYROID GLAND.
Four tiny bodies on the back of the thyroid gland, which is located in the neck. An important function of the parathyroid glands is to regulate the use of calcium and phosphorus in the body.

PAROTID GLANDS (also see: Mouth; Mumps; Tongue; etc.): The salivary glands found in front of, and below, the (outer) ear. They are shaped like small bunches of grapes.

Foot points: Palate (?).

PELVIS: The bony ring formed by the hip bones, the sacrum, the coccyx and the cavity formed by them.

Foot points: (?) Appendix; Prostate; Groin; Colon (all).

PERINEUM: That area of the body located between the anus and the sex organs.

Foot points: (?) Rectum; Sex organs.

PERIODONTAL PROBLEMS (e.g., pyorrhea, etc. — also see: Gingivitis; MOUTH; Toothache; etc.): Problems (e.g., inflammation, degeneration, etc.) of the gums, bone surrounding the teeth.

Foot points: Tooth, teeth; Palate.

PERITONITIS (also see: Abdomen, lower; etc.): An inflammation of the wall of the abdominal cavity resulting from any number of sources such as a ruptured appendix or wound, etc. Its symptoms include severe abdominal pain (often intensified by movement) and abdominal distention. Vomiting and/or diarrhea may be present in the early stages; fever, chills, and rapid pulse usually follow. The sufferer appears very sick — which he is.

Peritonitis is a complication of an underlying problem or condition; foods and fluids should not be given. This is an extremely serious problem and, untreated, will usually lead to death. Get medical help immediately.

Foot points: (?) Ileo-cecum; Prostate; Bladder (urinary); Appendix; Ureter tubes.

PHARYNX (also see: Larynx; RESPIRATORY SYSTEM;
Throat; Tonsillitis; etc.): The tube that runs from the
back of the nose to the esophagus.

Foot points: Throat; Thyroid; Tonsils.

PINEAL GLAND (also see: Brain; Endocrine glands; Head;
etc.): A pea-sized gland located near lower part of the
brain. While its function is not completely
understood, at least one part of its purpose is to deal
with the sex organs, their size and development. Like
all endocrine glands, its stimulation should only be
undertaken with great caution. (Note: Most schools of
yoga place high importance on this gland in terms of
spiritual and emotional development.)

Foot points: Pineal.

PITUITARY GLAND (also see: Endocrine glands; etc.):
A vital endocrine gland located near — and attached to
— the brain. Like many other endocrine glands, its
function is only partially understood. It is a master
control for the body's internal secretions (hormones)
and is at least partially responsible for sex
functions, growth, sexual development, defenses
against emergencies and diseases, etc. Stimulate
this gland with acupressure cautiously, if at all.

Foot points: Pituitary.

PLEURISY (also see: Chest; Pain control centers; Pneumonia; etc.): An inflammation of the inner chest cavity sometimes accompanying infections of the lungs and/or chest areas. The primary symptom is pain, either mild or severe, while breathing. Pleurisy is generally symptomatic of a more serious underlying conditon. Get medical help immediately.

Foot points: Lungs; Diaphragm.

PNEUMONIA (also see: Chest; Pleurisy; etc.): An inflammation of the air sacs in the lungs. There are a number of forms of pneumonia, and each represents a potentially dangerous threat. Often pneumonia is a complication of other problems or diseases. Colds and influenza, chronic alcoholism, malnutrition, exposure, and foreign matter in the respiratory tract are only a few of the conditions that may lead to this disorder.
   Although pneumonia may be either bacterial or non-bacterial, symptoms are the same and include shaking chills, sharp pain in either or both sides of the chest, cough with a pinkish-to-rusty sputum, fever and headache. Get medical help immediately.

Foot points: (?) Bronchial tubes; Lungs.

PROSTATE (also see: Sexual organs; etc.): The organ surrounding the neck of the urinary bladder in the male. Symptoms of prostate problems often include itching and burning in and around the front of the urethral canal (urethral meatus) of the penis, especially in the morning, and pain in the groin and/or lower back region.

Foot points: Prostate; Bladder, (urinary — ?).

PSORIASIS (also see: SKIN; etc.): A chronic, inflammatory skin and scalp disorder characterized by reddened patches covered with silvery white scales. This disorder tends to run in families and usually occurs after a strep infection, skin injury, emotional shock or stressful situation. It is not contagious, infectious or particularly uncomfortable. It is more common in people who drink large amounts of liquor.

Foot points: See SKIN.

RECTUM (also see: Gastrointestinal system; Gonorrhea; Hemorrhoids; etc.): The lowest part of the large intestine, ending at the anus.

Foot points: Rectum.

RESPIRATORY SYSTEM (also see: Bronchitis; Chest; Lungs; Pneumonia; etc.): The system of the body pertaining to the breathing apparatus. This includes the nasal cavities; pharynx; larynx; trachea; bronchi; broncheoles; and the lungs (primary organs, in traditional Oriental theory, which are paired with the colon).
   The most common problem to this system — and one of man's most common health problems — is the "common" cold (upper respiratory infection). Other problems include: Pneumonia; tuberculosis; emphysema; allergic reactions (e.g., "hay fever," sneezing, coughing, etc.); and, less commonly, such problems as celiac disease ("sprue" or gluten allergy), etc.

Foot points: Adrenals; Colon; Lungs.

RETCHING: See VOMITING AND RETCHING.

RHEUMATISM: See bodily area affected, such as Shoulder, etc.

RHINITIS: See Allergies; Hay fever; Nasal congestion; Sinusitis.

SCAPULA (shoulder blade — also see: Back, upper; etc.): The large triangular bones located in the upper back, to either side of the spine.

Foot points: See BACK, UPPER.

SCIATICA (also see: Back, lower; Buttocks; HIP; NEURALGIA; Leg; Lumbago; Pain control centers; etc.): Pain and tenderness along the sciatic nerve, ranging from the lower back down (distally) as far as the hand. Sciatica differs from "normal" back pain in that the pain usually radiates from the lower back down the rear portion of the leg (vs. being localized in the back alone).

Foot points: (?) Sciatic nerve; Hip; Nerves.

SEASICKNESS (also see: Travel sickness; Vertigo; Vomiting and retching; etc.): A minor-to-severe feeling of illness, nausea and queasiness, often accompanied by vomiting and retching, dizziness, loss of appetite, etc. It is primarily associated with the motion of a boat or ship at sea, but may be triggered by the rocking of an unstable platform.

continued next page...

While this unpleasant condition might last as long
as several days in an unstable site, it is usually only
a temporary problem that eases as one's equilibrium
becomes more attuned to the surrounding environment or
as soon as one reaches a firm, stable location. Drink
no alcohol. In traditional Oriental theory, seasickness
— and other forms of motion illness — are symptoms of
liver disorder (which helps explain why seasick
sufferers actually turn greenish — one indication of
extreme liver and/or gallbladder distress). Seasickness
is more prevalent during the day — especially on foggy
days — than at night.

Foot points (?) Liver; Gallbladder.

SEXUAL DRIVE (also see: FRIGIDITY; Genitourinary
system; IMPOTENCE; Sexual organs; etc.): Problems with
the sexual drive (libido or primal-pleasure drive) are
of one of two types: Being "too hot"; or being "too
cold."

"Too hot" is characterized by strong interest in or
aversion to sexual activity, to the point that it
becomes a problem (e.g., too much activity, thought
and/or fantasy directed toward sexual fullment, real or
imagined, on a regular basis). This is caused primarily
by "extreme" foods.

"Too cold" is characterized by little or no interest
in sexual activity, impotence, etc., which is generally
caused by disease (e.g., diabetes), drugs (e.g.,
certain hypertensives, etc.) or such dietary problems
as malnutrition, alcoholism, etc). Sexual drive is
primarily a "child" of the kidneys, liver and heart.
Any problems with these organs may reflect themselves
in the sexual drive.

continued next page...

Further information about "balancing" the sexual drive may be found in this author's HOW TO ENJOY SEX MORE WITH ACUGENICS (available through the G-Jo Institute).

Foot points: See FRIGIDITY; IMPOTENCE.

SEXUAL ORGANS (also see: GENITOURINARY SYSTEM; Sexual drive; Vaginitis; Gonorrhea; Prostate; etc.): Includes the penis, testicles and related parts of the male reproductive system; and the vagina, ovaries, and womb (uterus) of the female system. The sexual organs develop from — and are "children" of — the kidneys (and urinary bladder) in traditional Oriental theory.
   Common problems of the sexual organs include: Gonorrhea (see GONORRHEA); herpes simplex II virus (see HERPES...); vaginal yeast infections (see VAGINITIS); infections; pain in/around sexual organs; sterility/infertility (see FERTILITY); discharges; slow maturity; etc.

Foot points: Ovary; Sex organs; Ureter tubes.

SHINGLES (HERPES ZOSTER — also see: Bodily area affected): A particularly painful infection of the central nervous system. Its symptoms include small eruptions and neuralgic pain, especially around the waist. Shingles most often occurs in persons over fifty-years-old.

Foot points: (?) Umbilicus; Solar plexus.

SHOULDER (also see: NECK, etc.):

Foot points: Shoulder.

-81-

SINUSITIS (problems of the sinuses — also see: Headache; Nasal congestion; etc.): Inflammation of the sinus cavities in and around the nose and eyes. When an acupressure point is stimulated, there may be drainage. Sinusitis is an allergic reaction — much like hay fever (allergic rhinitis) — that is "triggered" by certain dietary, emotional and/or environmental phenomena but whose "stage is set" by continued abusive practices (usually dietary). It is primarily a problem of the kidneys, adrenals, lungs and colon (large intestine) in traditional Oriental theory. It may also be related to thyroid dysfunction and/or tooth infection.

Foot points: (?) Lungs; Nose; Sinuses; Kidneys; Adrenals.

SKIN (also see: Acne; etc.): In traditional Oriental theory, the skin is a "child" of the lungs and colon. A problem of the skin often also indicates an imbalanced state with the kidneys. Conversely, as the kidneys and/or lungs and colon return to balance, the skin clears. Skin problems may also indicate a thyroid dysfunction.

Foot points: Lungs; Colon; Kidneys; Bladder (urinary); Adrenals; Thyroid;

SMALL INTESTINE (also see: GASTROINTESTINAL SYSTEM; HEART; Ulcers, digestive; etc.): The primary organ — "mated" with heart, in traditional Oriental theory — which connects the bottom of the stomach with the beginning of the colon (large intestine).

continued next page...

The small intestine has three parts — the duodenum, the jejunum and ileum — and serves, among others, the functions of creating sludge from the stomach contents and several blood-related chores. (For more in-depth techniques for healing this organ, see this author's THE NATURAL HEALER'S ACUPRESSURE HANDBOOK, VOLUME II.)

Foot points: Intestine, small; Heart (?).

SNORING: During sleep, breathing in such a way as to rattle and vibrate the soft palate (usually when sleeping on back). May arise from "sleep apnea" (or "forgetting" to breathe for prolonged periods of time), and is most common in overweight males with short necks. (Note: Have victim — the person kept awake — try triggering points gently when snorer is snoring.)

Foot points: (?) Palate.

SOLAR PLEXUS (celiac plexus): The region — especially the nerve network — extending downward from the area of the heart into the upper abdomen.

Foot points: Solar plexus.

SORES (on skin — also see: Boils, styes, carbuncles; Skin; etc.): Skin disorders and eruptions, these are often symptoms of genitourinary disorder. Any slow-healing, returning or otherwise suspicious sore — especially on the face, ears, hands, lower forearms and/or lower legs (common sites for skin cancer to develop) — should have prompt medical attention.

Foot points: Use corresponding bodily area points.

SORE THROAT: See Colds and influenza; Throat; etc.

SPASM, MUSCULAR: See Cramps and spasms, muscular; Muscles; Pain control centers.

SPINAL CORD (also see: Back, lower and upper; Nerves; Vertebrae; etc.): That part of the central nervous system carried within the vertebral column (spine).

Foot points: (?) Nerves; Vertebrae (all).

SPLEEN (also see: Diabetes mellitus; Gallbladder; Liver; Pancreas; Stomach; etc.): Located in the upper left-hand quarter of the abdomen, beneath or behind the left side of the ribcage, the spleen is the largest lymph gland of the body. In traditional Oriental theory, it is paired with or "mated" (along with the pancreas) to the stomach and is a primary organ. The spleen is the central organ of the lymph system, whose chore is (among other functions) the cleansing of impurities from the blood.
    Splenic problems may manifest themselves as pain in the left side radiating up to the shoulder, hot and dry skin, thirst, possibly dark and scanty urine, constipation, etc. It is the primary organ affected by diabetes, in the traditional Oriental theory.
    The spleen is also vital in the process of controlling disease. Because of its close connection with the lymph system, it is important in the blood-cleansing and circulating process. Thus it is a primarily affected organ in such disorders as: Hodgkin's disease; leukemia; anemia; septicemia; etc.

continued next page...

The spleen is subject to such phenomena as enlargement or rupture as well as inflammation. In Western medical theory, the spleen is not considered essential and is removed by surgery regularly; in traditional Oriental theory, on the other, it is one of the five most important organs and is responsible for many functions of maintenance, both physical and emotional. (For more in-depth techniques for healing this organ, see this author's THE NATURAL HEALER'S ACUPRESSURE HANDBOOK, VOLUME II.)

Foot points: Spleen; Stomach; Pancreas; E-8; F-8; I-8; J-8.

SPRAINS, MUSCULAR (also see: Muscles; Pain control centers; Strains, muscular; specific areas of injury, such as Hand, Wrist, etc.): Injuries to the soft tissues surrounding the joints. Sprains generally occur when the joint is forced into more extreme action than it is capable of handling. Keep stress away from the sprained area since the injury is sometimes a tearing or partial ripping of the ligaments, muscles and/or blood vessels of the affected area.

Foot points: Use corresponding bodily area points.

STOMACH (also see: Abdomen, upper; Gallbladder; Gastrointestinal system; etc.): This dilated organ of the gastrointestinal system is located directly below the diaphragm. In traditional Oriental theory, the stomach is the organic "mate" of the spleen (and pancreas), and is a primary organ of digestion whose major physical function is breaking down and dissolving food.

continued on next page...

(Note: Pain arising soon after eating usually indicates trouble in upper stomach — especially a stomach ulcer — and is usually caused by excessive sweet/sugary foods; pain that is relieved by eating may indicate a duodenal ulcer. For more in-depth techniques for healing this organ, see this author's THE NATURAL HEALER'S ACUPRESSURE HANDBOOK, VOLUME II.)

Foot points: See GASTROINTESTINAL SYSTEM; Spleen (?); Pancreas (?); Stomach.

STONES, GALLBLADDER: See GALLSTONES.

STONES, KIDNEY or BLADDER (urolithiases — also see GENITOURINARY SYSTEM; KIDNEYS; etc.): Calculi formed from normal constituents of urine which have combined into a relatively insoluble crystalline substance by whatever deficiencies or imbalances that exist to precipitate them. There are several different kinds of kidney stones. May be associated with gout and symptomatic of incomplete protein absorption or assimilation. Kidney stones occur equally between both sexes, while bladder stones are far more frequent in males. Pain is likely to be excruciating — esp. in the flanks (area between ribs and hips) — if the stone(s) pass from the kidneys. Get medical help immediately. And since stones are of several types, if it passes out of the system, collect it for laboratory examination.

Foot points: (?) Ureter tubes; Kidneys; Bladder (urinary).

STRAINS, MUSCULAR (including "charley horse" — also
see: Muscles; Pain control centers; Sprains, muscular;
etc.): Muscular strains are much like sprains, except
they usually occur away from the joint. With muscular
strains, muscle fibers are stretched too far, sometimes
even torn. Strains commonly occur in the lower back,
triggered by improper lifting or hoisting. In short,
they are muscle injuries due to improper or over-
exertion.

Foot points: Use corresponding bodily area points.

STYES: See BOILS, STYES, AND CARBUNCLES.

SWELLING (also see: Edema; Sprains, muscular; Strains,
muscular; etc.): A non-specific accumulation of fluid
in various tissues. Since swelling without injury may
be symptomatic of potentially serious underlying health
problems, get medical attention for this problem.

Foot points: Use corresponding bodily area points.

TENNIS ELBOW: See ELBOW.

TESTICLES, INCLUDING CRUSHED TESTICLES (also see:
Pain control centers; Sexual organs; etc.): Injury to
the testicles is one of the most painful and agonizing
conditions that can happen to the male body; even a
mild injury to the testicles may be completely
debilitating.

Foot points: Sex organs.

TETANUS (lockjaw — also see: Bites, animal, human and insect: An infectious disease caused by a wound not exposed to oxygen. Any wound may result in tetanus infection; punctures and bites are notorious, especially where there is the presence of rust and/or fecal matter.

As tetanus progresses, spasms of the voluntary muscles occur and convulsions become frequent. Muscle stiffness after a puncture wound (any time between two and 50 days, but usually between five and 10 days) should lead you to suspect tetanus, especially if you have had no inoculation against the disease within several years.

With tetanus, the jaw muscles will eventually lock, accompanied by a grotesque grimace or smile with raised eyebrows. Untreated tetanus is generally fatal. For any wound, if you have not had a recent tetanus vaccination, get medical help immediately.

Foot points: Use corresponding bodily area points; Nerves.

THROAT (also see: Colds and influenza; Hoarseness; Laryngitis; Larynx; PHARYNX; RESPIRATORY SYSTEM; Tonsillitis; etc.): In traditional Oriental theory, the throat is primarily associated with the lungs and colon, and secondarily with the kidneys and urinary bladder.

Foot points: Throat; Lungs (?); Larynx.

THYMUS GLAND (also see: Endocrine glands; etc.): An endocrine gland, located in the chest near the heart. It is normal for this gland to be most active during the first year of life, then to atrophy to virtual non-existence. However, its effects are apparently felt throughout life, affecting primarily the sex glands, metabolism of calcium and in early years, the development of the skeleton. (Note: Any self-treatment of the endocrine glands should be done with moderation, if at all.)

Foot points: (?) Thymus.

THYROID GLAND (including Parathyroid gland — also see: Endocrine glands; Pharynx; etc.): One of the most vital endocrine glands, problems of the thyroid — which is located in the front part of the throat, along the windpipe (pharynx) — are often associated with diabetic or pre-diabetic conditions. Other conditions reflected/caused by dysfunctioning thyroid include: Goiter; certain heart disorders; "pop-eyed" (Graves) disease; cretinism; etc.
    Common symptoms of imbalanced thyroid activity include: Cold feet; low energy; poor growth (in children); arrhythmia; sexual difficulties; heat intolerance; dry skin; chapped lips; coarse skin; nervousness; weight imbalances; goiter; etc. (Note: Any self-treatment of the endocrine glands should be done with moderation, if at all.)

Foot points: Thyroid (and parathyroid); Throat.

TINNITUS (also see: EAR; HEARING DIFFICULTIES; etc.):
A disorder of the inner ear characterized by a ringing
sensation, often coupled with dizziness, may be a
result of high blood pressure, glandular disorder, ear
wax, etc. Often a symptom of Meniere's Syndrome.

Foot points: Ear; Kidneys; Bladder (urinary);
Eustachian tubes.

TONGUE (also see: MOUTH; Tonsillitis; etc.): In
traditional Oriental theory, the tongue — which
functions as the primary "sub-organ" of taste, speech
and swallowing — is a "child" of the heart and is
also closely associated with the stomach. Thus,
ailments of the tongue may indicate imbalance of one
or both those major organs.

Foot points: Tongue.

TONSILLITIS (also see: Throat; Pancreas; Pharynx;
SPLEEN; Stomach; etc.): Inflammation of the tonsils
(small glands in the throat). Symptoms include
chills, soreness, rapidly rising temperature, difficulty in swallowing, stiff neck, etc.
    In traditional Oriental theory, the tonsils are
related to the spleen (and pancreas). Abuses to these
organs quickly "reflect" themselves in inflammation of
the tonsils (if you are prone to tonsillitis). (Note:
After tonsillectomies — removal of tonsils — people
run a higher risk of lymph cancer — called Hodgkin's
Disease — and multiple sclerosis. On the other hand,
complications of tonsillitis may include scarlet fever,
sinusitis, ear infections, quinsy — a peritonsillar
abscess — and, rarely, arthritis or meningitis.)

Foot points: Throat; Tonsils.

TOOTH, TEETH (including GUMS — also see: Dental
Work; Jaw, lower, upper; MOUTH; TOOTHACHE; etc.):
In traditional Oriental theory, the teeth are
considered primarily as "children" of the colon
(large intestine).

Common problems of the teeth and gums include:
Decay (cavities or dental caries); spongy gums;
receding gums; infection and toothache; bruxism (or
tooth-grinding, esp. during sleep). Cavities and
pyorrhea (a gum disease) seldom occur in the same
mouth.

Foot points: Tooth, teeth; Palate (?).

TOOTHACHE (also see: DENTAL WORK; TOOTH,
TEETH, etc.): Pain in the nerve of a tooth, usually
caused by infection or inflammation arising from dental
caries (cavities). Since gums are essential parts of
the tooth system, a problem in these soft tissues which
cover the alveolar bone may also be the source of tooth
problems.

Abscesses (pods of infection, usually at the bases
of teeth) may directly or indirectly affect the heart,
lungs, liver, gallbladder, stomach or kidneys (at
least) — usually depending on the specific tooth
affected — so it is important to seek prompt
medical/dental attention for any toothache.

Foot points: (?) Throat; Tooth, teeth.

TOOTH EXTRACTION, DRILLING, etc.: See DENTAL
WORK.

TORTICOLLIS (stiff neck, "wry neck"): See NECK;
WHIPLASH (neck injury).

TRACHEA (also see: Larynx; Respiratory system;
Throat; etc.): The windpipe extending from the larynx
to the bronchi.

Foot points: Trachea.

TRAVEL SICKNESS (also see: Seasickness; Vertigo;
etc.): A general term for the symptoms that arise from
motion and instability. The inner ear and the liver
are the primarily affected bodily area and organ.

Foot points: See SEASICKNESS.

"TRAVELER'S DIARRHEA": A mild-to-moderate form of
amebic dysentery often encountered when traveling in
warm, primitive countries.

Foot points: See DYSENTERY.

TRIGEMINAL NEURALGIA (tic doloureaux — also see:
Face; Nerves; Neuralgia; etc.): A particularly painful
form of facial neuralgia that generally begins in
middle life and occurs more frequently in females than
males. Both the intensity of pain and frequency (as
well as duration) of attacks tend to increase. Seizures
appear to occur more frequently in spring and fall as
well as near the changes of season.

Foot points: (?) Ear; Neck; Nerves: Throat.

ULCERS (digestive — also see: Abdomen, upper; GASTROINTESTINAL SYSTEM; Stomach; etc.): Lesions that form in the digestive tract, often associated with stress. There are several types, depending in which section of the gastrointestinal system they form:
1. Stomach (gastric) ulcer — characterized by a "sluggish" stomach (from underproduction of stomach acids) that is aggravated by eating;
2. Intestinal (duodenal) ulcers — characterized by "hunger" pains that are relieved — and stay relieved for several hours — by eating.

Ulcer symptoms tend to peak in spring and fall, with bleeding from an ulcer being most common in January and September.

Foot points: See GASTROINTESTINAL SYSTEM.

ULCERS, ORAL ("thrush," canker sores, "trench mouth," etc. — also see: MOUTH; etc.): Lesions which develop from fungus infections, ususally in infants or elderly people. These are often accompanied by fever, gastrointestinal distress and the infection may spread to other parts of the body (e.g., buttocks, groin, etc.).

Foot points: See MOUTH.

ULCERS, SKIN (also see: Diabetes; SKIN; Varicose veins; etc.): Nearly always, ulcers (and similar lesions) of the skin arise from an underlying health problem (e.g., diabetes mellitus, varicose veins, etc.). Get immediate medical attention for any ulceration (or similar deep sores) of the skin.

Foot points: See SKIN.

URETERS, URETER TUBES (also see: Bladder, urinary; GENITOURINARY SYSTEM; Kidneys; etc.): The long, slender tubes leading/carrying urine from the kidneys to the urinary bladder.

Foot points: See GENITOURINARY SYSTEM; Ureter tubes.

URETHRA (also see: Bladder, urinary; GENITOURINARY SYSTEM; etc.): The tube (longer on males, shorter in females) leading from the urinary bladder to carry urine out of the body. (Note: Any urethritis — infection of the urethra — may be symptomatic of a venereal disease, such as gonorrhea, etc.; if this is suspected, get medical help immediately.)

Foot points: See GENITOURINARY SYSTEM.

URINARY CONTROL CENTERS (also see: Cystitis; Genitourinary system; Stones, kidney or bladder; etc.): To help bring temporary relief (up to half an hour or so) from the need to urinate. This technique may be helpful in a situation where facilities are not immediately available, as in driving, etc.
Frequent urination (more than six times daily for a male or seven times daily for a female) on a prolonged basis (beyond a short stressful period in life, say) may require professional attention.

Foot points: Bladder (urinary); Kidneys (?); Prostate (?).

UTERUS (womb — also see GENITOURINARY SYSTEM; Sexual organs; etc.): The three-inch long, thick walled female reproductive organ that receives and holds the (fertilized) egg which develops into the fetus. If the egg is not fertilized, then the lining is shed each month (menstruation).

Foot points: See GENITOURINARY SYSTEM; SEX ORGANS.

VAGINITIS (vaginal yeast infection, etc. — also see: Cystitis; GENITOURINARY SYSTEM; Sexual organs; etc.): A very common female ailment sometimes transmitted by males through sexual intercourse. Its symptoms — commonly abnormal itching, burning, discharge, etc. — may mask more serious problems, especially syphilis, gonorrhea, etc. For this reason — and because your sexual partner(s) may need treatment — seek medical advice if this condition is suspected.

Yeast (candida, monilia) is a common cause of vaginitis, as are trichomonas and other parasites or bacteria. Diabetes, pregnancy and taking birth control pills are also important possible factors in this condition.

The following "self-diagnosis" may be helpful in identifying the type of vaginal infection you are suffering:

Yeast — produces thick, white, creamy and/or curd-like discharge (usually odorless but with intense itching and/or burning/soreness). This condition often occurs in pregnancy and diabetes as a result of contraceptives, etc.

Bacterial — produces a watery, gray-to-white discharge that may by foul-smelling, but is seldom accompanied by much physical discomfort.

continued next page...

<u>Non-Specific</u> — produces a foul-smelling discharge (and may arise from a combination of bacteria). (Note: Vaginitis may be a symptom of gonorrhea or other sexually transmittable disease — if this is suspected, get medical help immediately).

<u>Foot points:</u> See GENITOURINARY SYSTEM; Sex organs.

VARICOSE VEINS: Swollen, inflamed/enlarged veins, most often found on the inner and/or back side of the calf and inner thigh. They are most often the shallower (vs. deeper) veins — those which are less supported by muscles.
    Varicose veins may be caused by such problems as phlebitis, pregnancy (or other excessive weight/ pressure on the abdomen), etc. Ulceration may occur in advanced cases. (Note: Varicose veins may be a precursor of thrombo-phlebitis — a dangerous condition; get medical attention for any varicose veins, or for symptoms of aching, burning, itching and/or pain, especially in the legs.)

<u>Foot points:</u> Liver; Kidneys.

VERTEBRAE/S (also see: Back, lower and/or upper; etc.): The 33 bones forming the vertebral (spinal) column. This column is "divided" into "sections": <u>Cervical</u> (highest — from the head to the shoulder area); <u>Thoracic</u> (central — from the top rib to the lowest rib); <u>Lumbar</u> (lower — from the bottom rib downward); <u>Sacral</u> (<u>sacrum</u> — the triangular "bone" at the bottom of the spine, just above the coccyx, comprised of five fused vertebrae).

<u>Foot points:</u> Vertebrae, cervical, lumbar, sacral, thoracic.

VERTIGO (also see: Seasickness; Travel sickness; etc.):
True vertigo is a sensation/ feeling that the outer
world is revolving about the sufferer (as may occur
with intoxication) or that he himself is moving in some
disoriented space. However, vertigo is more commonly
(and erroneously) used to mean dizziness, giddiness,
lightheadedness, etc. Vertigo may also be accompanied
by ringing in the ears (tinnitus) and/or rapid,
uncontrolled eye movements (nystagmus).

Foot points: See SEASICKNESS.

VITILIGO (also see: SKIN; etc.): A disorder of the skin
pigmentation in which pigmentation (skin coloring)
disappears, leaving spots or patches of white. While
spontaneous repigmentation may occur, it is rare. The
disorder is probably related to a dysfunction of the
lungs and/or kidneys (in traditional Oriental theory).

Foot points: Use corresponding bodily area points (?).

VOMITING AND RETCHING (also see: Stomach; etc.):
Symptomatic of many problems, and not all of them
associated with the digestive tract. Dehydration is
always a problem with continued loss of fluids; if
vomiting is severe, get medical help immediately.
Note: It is vital to prevent dehydration, especially
in the very young, the elderly and the seriously ill or
injured.

Feed Gatorade® or similar fluid replacer — if not available, use one qt. of boiled water plus juice of four oranges plus seven tsp. of white sugar plus one tsp. of salt; sip, medicinally. Also, if there is repeated vomiting/nausea after head injury, medical attention is imperative.

Foot points: Stomach; Diaphragm.

WHIPLASH (neck injury — also see: Neck; Pain control centers; etc.): A condition that may occur when the neck is snapped suddenly forward or back, as in the event of an automobile accident. Get medical help immediately.

Foot points: (?) Neck.

How to Heal Yourself Using Foot Acupressure (Foot Reflexology)

Section II:

Foot Acupressure Points and Their Illustrated Locations

REMINDER: The acupressure points in the following pages are approximate. They represent a compilation of the opinions of many authorities in the field of acupressure plus the author's own experience. The precise location of your own points will be determined by finding the most pressure-sensitive spots in the general areas described and illustrated in the following pages.

ALSO: In the following pages you may find an acupressure point preceded — or followed — by a question mark (?). This is meant to indicate an unacknowledged (by other authorities in the field) but probable location, based on the author's experience and/or acupressure theory.

FOOT ACUPRESSURE POINTS AND
THEIR ILLUSTRATED LOCATIONS

NAME OF FOOT POINT	LOCATION OF FOOT POINT
Adrenals	C-9, 10, 11; D-8, 9, 10; E-7; J-7, 8, 9, 10; K-7, 8, 9, 10, 12; L-11, 12
Ankle	C-15, 16; D-15, 16; K-15, 16; L-15, 16
Anus	D-17; E-17; J-16, 17; K-17
Appendix	B-15; C-12, 13, 14, 15
Arm	A-7, 8, 9, 10, 11, 12; M-13, 14, 15; N-6, 7, 8, 9, 10, 11, 12, 13, 14
Bladder (urinary)	E-14, 15, 16; F-9, 10, 11; I-9, 10, 11, 12; J-11, 12, 13, 14

Brain	A-3; B-1; C-1; D-1; E-1; F-1; G-1; H-1; I-1; J-1; K-1; L-1; M-1, 3; N-3
Breast	B-6; C-6; L-6, 7; M-6
Bronchial tubes	C-5, 6; D-5, 6; E-5, 6; J-5, 6; K-5, 6; L-5
Coccyx	E-16, 17; J-16, 17; K-17
Colon (general)	D-17; E-17; J-16
Colon, ascending	B-12, 13, 14, 15; C-10, 11, 12, 13, 14, 15, 16
Colon, descending	L-10, 11, 12, 13, 14, 15, 16; M-13, 14, 15
Colon, Sigmoid	See Sigmoid colon, flexure
Colon, transverse	D-10, 12, 13; E-10, 13; F-10; I-9, 10; J-10, 13; K-10, 13, 14; L-10, 13, 14
Diaphragm	C-7, 10; D-7, 9, 10; E-7; J-7; K-7, 11; L-7, 8, 9
Ear	A-5; B-4, 5; C-3, 4; M-4, 5; N-5
Elbow	A-11; N-10, 11
Epiglottis	G-7; H-7
Eustachian tubes	A-4; B-5; M-4; N-5

Eye	D-3, 4; E-4; F-4; I-4, 5; J-4, 5 K-4; L-4
Foot, feet	C-15, 16; D-15, 16; K-15, 16; L-15, 16
Gallbladder	C-8, 9; D-11;
Heart	J-8; K-8, 9; L-6, 7;
Hip	B-16, 17; M-16, 17; N-14;
Ileo-cecum	B-15; C-11, 12, 13, 14, 15
Intestine, small	C-11, 12, 13, 14, 15; D-11, 14, 15, 16; E-11, 14, 15, 16; J-10, 11, 12, 13, 14, 15; K-10, 11, 12, 13, 14, 15, 16; L-10, 11, 14, 15
Kidneys	C-6, 7, 8, 12; D-6, 7, 8, 9, 10, 11, 12; E-9; J-9; K-6, 7, 8, 9, 10, 11, 12, 13; L-6, 7, 8, 12, 13;
Knee	B-12, 13, 14, 15; M-12, 13, 14, 15; N-12, 13, 14
Larynx	G-6, 7; H-5, 6
Liver	B-8, 11; C-8, 9, 11; D-8, 9
Lungs	C-5, 6, 7, 8, 9, 10; D-5, 6, 7, 8, 9; E-5, 6, 7, 8; J-5, 6, 7, 8, 9, 10; K-5, 6, 7, 8, 9, 10, 11; L-5, 6, 7, 8, 9

Lymph nodes, drainage	B-6; C-6; L-6; M-6;
Neck	F-4; G-3, 4; H-4; I-4
Nerves	C-6; D-6, 7; E-7; I-7; J-7; K-7; L-6
Nose	G-2, 3, 4, 5; H-2, 3, 4, 5;
Ovary	C-16, 17; D-17; K-16, 17; L-17
Palate	F-5; G-5
Pancreas	D-8, 9; E-8, 9, 10; I-8,9; J-8, 9, 10; L-10; M-10
Pineal gland	F-2, 3; G-2, 3; H-2, 3; I-2, 3
Pituitary gland	F-2, 3; G-2, 3; H-2, 3; I-2, 3
Prostate	E-17; J-16, 17; K-17
Rectum	D-17; E-17; J-16;
Sciatic nerve	B-16, 17; L-17; M-16, 17
Sex organs	D-17; E-16, 17; J-16, 17; K-17
Shoulder	A-6; B-5, 6; C-3; K-3; L-3, 4; M-5, 6; N-6
Sigmoid colon, flexure	J-14, 15, 16; K-14, 15, 16; L-14, 15, 16

Sinuses	A-3, 4, 5; B-1, 2, 3, 4, 5; C-1, 2, 3, 4; D-1, 2, 3, 4; E-1, 2, 3, 4; F-1, 2, 3, 4; I-2, 3, 5; J-1, 2, 3, 4, 5; K-1, 2, 3, 4; L-1, 2, 3, 4; M-1, 2, 3, 4, 5; N-4, 5
Solar plexus	C-7; D-7; E-7; J-7; K-7, 9; L-7, 8
Spleen	L-8, 9, 10, 11; M-10, 11
Stomach	D-6, 7, 11; E-6, 7, 11; F-6, 7; H-6, 7; I-6, 7, 8; J-6, 7, 8, 11; K-7, 8, 12; L-7, 8
Throat	G-4; H-4; I-4;
Thymus	C-6, 7; D-6, 7; E-5; F-5; I-5; J-6, 7; K-6, 7
Thyroid and parathyroid	E-5, 6, 7, 8; F-5; G-4; H-4; I-5, 6; J-5, 6, 7, 8
Tongue	G-4, 5; H-3, 4, 5
Tonsils	F-4, 5; I-5; J-5, 6
Tooth; teeth	A-5; B-4, 5; C-3, 4; D-4; E-4; F-4; I-5; J-4, 5; K-4; L-4; M-4, 5; N-5
Trachea	G-6, 7; H-5, 6
Umbilicus	D-10; E-10; J-10; K-10

Ureter tubes	D-10, 11, 12, 13; E-12, 13; K-10, 11, 12, 13; L-13
Vertebrae, cervical	F-8; G-4, 5, 6; H-4, 5, 6
Vertebrae, lumbar	E-12; F-10, 11, 12; I-10, 11, 12; J-10, 11, 12
Vertebrae, sacral	E-12, 13, 15, 16; F-12; I-12; J-11, 13, 14, 15, 16
Vertebrae, thoracic	E-10, 11; F-9, 10, 11; G-5, 6, 7; H-5, 6, 7; I-8, 9, 10

NAME OF FOOT POINT: Adrenals

NAME OF FOOT POINT: C-9, 10, 11; D-8, 9, 10; E-7; J-7,
8, 9, 10; K-7, 8, 9, 10, 12; L-11, 12

NAME OF FOOT POINT: Ankle

LOCATION OF POINT: C-15, 16; D-15, 16; K-15, 16; L-15, 16

NAME OF FOOT POINT: Anus

NAME OF FOOT POINT: D-17; E-17; J-16, 17; K-17

NAME OF FOOT POINT: Appendix

LOCATION OF POINT: B-15; C-12, 13, 14, 15;

NAME OF FOOT POINT: Arm

LOCATION OF POINT: A-7, 8, 9, 10, 11, 12; M-13, 14, 15;
    N-6, 7, 8, 9, 10, 11, 12, 13, 14

NAME OF FOOT POINT: Bladder (urinary)

LOCATION OF POINT: E-14, 15, 16; F-9, 10, 11; I-9, 10, 11, 12; J-11, 12, 13, 14

NAME OF FOOT POINT: Brain

LOCATION OF POINT: A-3; B-1; C-1; D-1; E-1; F-1; G-1;
H-1; I-1; J-1; K-1; L-1; M-1, 3; N-3

NAME OF FOOT POINT: Breast

LOCATION OF POINT: B-6; C-6; L-6, 7; M-6;

NAME OF FOOT POINT: Bronchial tubes

LOCATION OF POINT: C-5, 6; D-5, 6; E-5, 6; J-5, 6; K-5, 6; L-5

Right Foot   Left Foot

NAME OF FOOT POINT: Coccyx

LOCATION OF POINT: E-16, 17; J-16, 17; K-17

NAME OF FOOT POINT: Colon (general)

LOCATION OF POINT: D-17; E-17; J-16;

NAME OF FOOT POINT: Colon, ascending

LOCATION OF POINT: B-12, 13, 14, 15; C-10, 11, 12, 13, 14, 15, 16

NAME OF FOOT POINT: Colon, descending

LOCATION OF POINT: L-10, 11, 12, 13, 14, 15, 16; M-13, 14, 15

NAME OF FOOT POINT: Colon, transverse

LOCATION OF POINT: D-10, 12, 13; E-10, 13; F-10; I-9, 10; J-10, 13; K-10, 13, 14; L-10, 13, 14

NAME OF FOOT POINT: Diaphragm

LOCATION OF POINT: C-7, 10; D-7, 9, 10; E-7; J-7; K-7, 11; L-7, 8, 9

NAME OF FOOT POINT: Ear

LOCATION OF POINT: A-5; B-4, 5; C-3, 4; M-4, 5; N-5

NAME OF FOOT POINT: Elbow

LOCATION OF POINT: A-11; N-10, 11;

NAME OF FOOT POINT: Epiglottis

LOCATION OF POINT: G-7; H-7,

NAME OF FOOT POINT: Eustachian tubes

LOCATION OF POINT: A-4; B-5; M-4; N-5;

NAME OF FOOT POINT: Eye

LOCATION OF POINT: D-3, 4; E-4; F-4; I-4, 5; J-4, 5
K-4; L-4

NAME OF FOOT POINT: Foot, feet

LOCATION OF POINT: C–15, 16; D–15, 16; K–15, 16; L–15, 16

NAME OF FOOT POINT: Gallbladder

LOCATION OF POINT: C-8, 9; D-11;

NAME OF FOOT POINT: Heart

LOCATION OF POINT: J-8; K-8, 9; L-6, 7;

NAME OF FOOT POINT: Hip

LOCATION OF POINT: B-16, 17; M-16, 17; N-14;

NAME OF FOOT POINT: Ileo-cecum

LOCATION OF POINT: B-15; C-11, 12, 13, 14, 15

NAME OF FOOT POINT: Intestine, small

LOCATION OF POINT: C-11, 12, 13, 14, 15; D-11, 14, 15, 16; E-11, 14, 15, 16; J-10, 11, 12, 13, 14, 15; K-10, 11, 12, 13, 14, 15, 16; L-10, 11, 14, 15

Right Foot   Left Foot

NAME OF FOOT POINT: Kidneys

LOCATION OF POINT: C-6, 7, 8, 12; D-6, 7, 8, 9, 10, 11,
    12; E-9; J-9; K-6, 7, 8, 9, 10, 11, 12, 13; L-6, 7,
    8, 12, 13

NAME OF FOOT POINT: Knee

LOCATION OF POINT: B-12, 13, 14, 15; M-12, 13, 14, 15;
   N-12, 13, 14

NAME OF FOOT POINT: Larynx

LOCATION OF POINT: G-6, 7; H-5, 6;

NAME OF FOOT POINT: Liver

LOCATION OF POINT: B–8, 11; C–8, 9, 11; D–8, 9;

NAME OF FOOT POINT: Lungs

LOCATION OF POINT: C-5, 6, 7, 8, 9, 10; D-5, 6, 7, 8, 9; E-5, 6, 7, 8; J-5, 6, 7, 8, 9, 10; K-5, 6, 7, 8, 9, 10, 11; L-5, 6, 7, 8, 9;

Right Foot   Left Foot

NAME OF FOOT POINT: Lymph nodes, drainage

LOCATION OF POINT: B-6; C-6; L-6; M-6;

NAME OF FOOT POINT: Neck

LOCATION OF POINT: F-4; G-3, 4; H-4; I-4

NAME OF FOOT POINT: Nerves

LOCATION OF POINT: C-6; D-6, 7: E-7; I-7; J-7; K-7; L-6

NAME OF FOOT POINT: Nose

LOCATION OF POINT: G-2, 3, 4, 5; H-2, 3, 4, 5;

NAME OF FOOT POINT: Ovary

LOCATION OF POINT: C-16, 17; D-17; K-16, 17; L-17;

NAME OF FOOT POINT: Palate

LOCATION OF POINT: F-5; G-5

NAME OF FOOT POINT: Pancreas

LOCATION OF POINT: D-8, 9; E-8, 9, 10; I-8, 9; J-8, 9,
    10; L-10; M-10;

NAME OF FOOT POINT: Pineal gland

LOCATION OF POINT: F-2, 3; G-2, 3; H-2, 3; I-2, 3

NAME OF FOOT POINT: Pituitary gland

LOCATION OF POINT: F-2, 3; G-2, 3; H-2, 3; I-2, 3

NAME OF FOOT POINT: Prostate

LOCATION OF POINT: E-17; J-16, 17; K-17

NAME OF FOOT POINT: Rectum

LOCATION OF POINT: D–17; E–17; J–16;

NAME OF FOOT POINT: Sciatic nerve

LOCATION OF POINT: B-16, 17; L-17; M-16, 17

NAME OF FOOT POINT: Sex organs

LOCATION OF POINT: D–17; E–16, 17; J–16, 17; K–17;

NAME OF FOOT POINT: Shoulder

LOCATION OF POINT: A-6; B-5, 6; C-3; K-3; L-3, 4; M-5, 6; N-6;

NAME OF FOOT POINT: Sigmoid colon, flexure

LOCATION OF POINT: J-14, 15, 16; K-14, 15, 16; L-14, 15, 16

NAME OF FOOT POINT: Sinuses

LOCATION OF POINT: A-3, 4, 5; B-1, 2, 3, 4, 5; C-1, 2,
3, 4; D-1, 2, 3, 4; E-1, 2, 3, 4; F-1, 2, 3, 4; I-2,
3, 5; J-1, 2, 3, 4, 5; K-1, 2, 3, 4; L-1, 2, 3, 4;
M-1, 2, 3, 4, 5; N-4, 5

NAME OF FOOT POINT: Solar plexus

LOCATION OF POINT: C-7; D-7; E-7; J-7; K-7, 9; L-7, 8

NAME OF FOOT POINT: Spleen

LOCATION OF POINT: L-8, 9, 10, 11; M-10, 11;

NAME OF FOOT POINT: Stomach

LOCATION OF POINT: D-6, 7, 11; E-6, 7, 11; F-6, 7; H-6, 7; I-6, 7, 8; J-6, 7, 8, 11; K-7, 8, 12; L-7, 8

Right Foot   Left Foot

NAME OF FOOT POINT: Throat

LOCATION OF POINT: G-4; H-4; I-4;

NAME OF FOOT POINT: Thymus

LOCATION OF POINT: C-6, 7; D-6, 7; E-5; F-5; I-5; J-6, 7; K-6, 7

NAME OF FOOT POINT: Thyroid and parathyroid

LOCATION OF POINT: E-5, 6, 7, 8; F-5; G-4; H-4; I-5, 6; J-5, 6, 7, 8

NAME OF FOOT POINT: Tongue

LOCATION OF POINT: G-4, 5; H-3, 4, 5;

NAME OF FOOT POINT: Tonsils

LOCATION OF POINT: F-4, 5; I-5; J-5, 6

NAME OF FOOT POINT: Tooth; teeth

LOCATION OF POINT: A-5; B-4, 5; C-3, 4; D-4; E-4; F-4; I-5; J-4, 5; K-4; L-4; M-4, 5; N-5

NAME OF FOOT POINT: Umbilicus

LOCATION OF POINT: D-10; E-10; J-10; K-10

NAME OF FOOT POINT: Trachea

LOCATION OF POINT: G-6, 7; H-5, 6

NAME OF FOOT POINT: Ureter tubes

LOCATION OF POINT: D-10, 11, 12, 13; E-12, 13; K-10, 11, 12, 13; L-13

NAME OF FOOT POINT: Vertebrae, cervical

LOCATION OF POINT: F-8; G-4, 5, 6; H-4, 5, 6

NAME OF FOOT POINT: Vertebrae, lumbar

LOCATION OF POINT: E-12; F-10, 11, 12; I-10, 11, 12;
J-10, 11, 12

NAME OF FOOT POINT: Vertebrae, sacral

LOCATION OF POINT: E-12, 13, 15, 16; F-12; I-12; J-11, 13, 14, 15, 16

NAME OF FOOT POINT: Vertebrae, thoracic

LOCATION OF POINT: E-10, 11; F-9, 10, 11; G-5, 6, 7; H-5, 6, 7; I-8, 9, 10

BIBLIOGRAPHY

The following publications have been helpful to the author and/or will be of interest for further studies by the reader.

Abrams, Albert, A.M., LL.D., M. New Concepts in Diagnosis and Treatment. Mokelumne Hill, CA: Health Research (reprint), P.O. Box 70, 1977.

Acupuncture Anaesthesia. Peking, China: Foreign Languages Press, 1972.

Austin, Dr. Mary. Acupuncture Therapy. New York: ASI Publishers, Inc. 1972.

Barefoot Doctor's Manual, A (N.I.H. 75-695). Superintendant of Documents, Washington, D.C. 20402.

Beau, Georges. Chinese Medicine. New York: Avon Books, 1972.

Blakiston's Pocket Medical Dictionary. New York: McGraw-Hill Book Co., third edition, 1972.

Carter, Mildred. Hand Reflexology: Key to Perfect Health. West Nyack, NY: Parker Publishing Co., Inc., 1975.

Carter, Mildred. Helping Yourself With Foot
Reflexology. West Nyack, NY: Parker Publishing Co.,
Inc., 1974.

Cerney, J. V., A.B., D.M., D.P.M. Acupuncture Without
Needles. West Nyack, NY: Parker Publishing Co.,
Inc., 1974.

Chan, Pedro, Ph.D. Ear Acupressure. Monterey Park,
CA: Chan's Corporation, P.O. Box 478, 1981.

Chan, Pedro, Finger Acupressure. Los Angeles:
Price/Stern/Sloan Publishers, 1974

Chan, Pedro. Wonders of Chinese Acupuncture.
Alhambra, CA: Borden Publishing Co., 1973.

Dale, Ralph A., Ph.D., Ed.D. Acupuncture with Your
Fingers. Surfside, FL: Dialectic Press, P.O. Box
6622, 1980.

Dale, Ralph A., Ph.D., Ed.D. Acupuncture in Physical
Therapy. Surfside, FL: Dialectic Press, 1981.

Dale, Ralph A., Ph.D., Ed.D. Microacupuncture Systems
(books One and Two). Surfside, FL: Dialectic Press,
1981.

Duke, Marc. Acupuncture. New York: Pyramid Books,
1972.

Hashimoto, Mme. Dr. M. Japanese Acupuncture. 91 St.
Martins Lane, London W.C.2, England: Thorson's
Publishers, Ltd., 1962.

Houston, F.M., D.C. The Healing Benefits of
Acupressure. New Canaan, CT.: Keats Publishing,
Inc., 1974.

Huang, Helena L., Ph.D. (translator) Ear Acupuncture.
Emmaus, PA: Rodale Press, 1974.

Ingham, Eunice D. Stories the Feet Can Tell.
Rochester, NY: Eunice D. Ingham, Box 948, 1959.

Ingham, Eunice D. Stories the Feet Have Told.
Rochester, NY: Eunice D. Ingham, 1959.

Jain, K.K., M.D. The Amazing Story of Health Care in
China. Emmaus, PA: Rodale Press, 1973.

Kao, Frederick F., editor. The American Journal of
Chinese Medicine. Volumes I, II, III, through number
3, July, 1975.

Kushi, Michio. Acupuncture, Ancient and Future
Worlds. Boston: East West Foundation, 1979.

Kushi, Michio. An Introduction to Oriental Diagnosis.
London: Red Moon Press; 12 Orpheus St., S.E.5, 1978.

Lavier, Dr. J. Points of Chinese Acupuncture
(translated, indexed, and adapted by Dr. Philip M.
Chancellor). Denington Estate, Wellingborough,
Northhamptonshire, England: Health Science Press,
second edition, 1974.

Lawson-Wood, D. & J. Acupuncture Handbook. England:
Health Science Press, second edition, 1973.

Lawson-Wood, D. & J. First Aid at Your Fingertips.
England: Health Science Press, 1963.

Lawson-Wood, D. & J. Five Elements of Acupuncture and Chinese Massage. England: Health Science Press, 1966.

Lawson-Wood, D. & J. Judo Revival Points, Athletes' Points and Posture. England: Health Science Press, 1960.

Lawson-Wood, D. & J. The Incredible Healing Needles. England: Health Science Press, 1974.

Lu, Henry, Ph.D. Chinese Acupressure. Vancouver, B.C., V6M 4G1, Canada: Academy of Oriental Heritage, P.O. Box 35057, Station E, 1977.

Lu, Henry, Ph.D. Chinese Diet for Your Health: Academy of Oriental Heritage, 1980.

Lu, Henry, Ph.D. Cook-it-yourself Chinese Health Foods: Academy of Oriental Heritage, 1977.

Lu, Henry, Ph.D. Introduction to Chinese Manipulative Therapy: Academy of Oriental Heritage, 1978.

Lu, Henry, Ph.D. Physicians' Guide to Dr. Lu's Chinese Diagnosis and Treatment Charts: Academy of Oriental Heritage, 1977.

Manaka, Dr. Y., and Urquhart, Dr. I. A. Chinese Massage. San Francisco: Japan Publications Trading Co., 1973.

Mann, Felix, M.B. Acupuncture, the Ancient Chinese Art of Healing. London: Wm. Heinemann Medical Books, Ltd., second edition, 1972.

Mann, Felix, M.B. Acupuncture, the Ancient Chinese Art of Healing and How It Works Scientifically. New York: Vintage Books (division of Random House)., 1973.

Mann, Felix, M.B. Acupuncture, Cure of Many Diseases. London: Wm. Heinemann Medical Books, Lte., 1971.

Mann, Felix, M.B. Atlas of Acupuncture. London: Wm. Heinemann Medical Books, Ltd., 1971.

Mann, Felix, M.B. The Meridians of Acupuncture. London: Wm. Heinemann Medical Books, Ltd., 1971.

Mann, Felix, M.B. The Treatment of Disease by Acupuncture. London: Wm. Heinemann Medical Books, Ltd., 1971.

Masunaga, Shizuto. Zen Shiatsu. San Francisco: Japan Publications Trading Co., 1977.

Matsumoto, Teruo, M.D., Ph.D., F.A.C.S. Acupuncture for Physicians. Springfield, IL: Charles C. Thomas, Publishers, 1974.

Merck Manual of Diagnosis and Therapy, The. Rahway, NJ: Merck & Co., Inc. eleventh edition, 1966.

McGarey, Wm. A., M.D. Acupuncture and Body Energies. Phoenix, AR: Gabriel Press, 1974.

Moss, Dr. Louis. Acupuncture and You. 2 All Saints St., London, N.1.: Elek Books, 1964.

Namikoshi, Tokujiro. Shiatsu: Health and Vitality at Your Fingertips. San Francisco: Japan Publications Trading Co., 1969.

Namikolshi, Toru. Shiatsu Therapy: Theory and
Practice. San Francisco: Japan Publications Trading
Co., 1977.

Ohashi, Wataru. Do-it-yourself Shiatsu. San
Francisco: Japan Publications Trading Co., 1976.

Ohsawa, George. Acupuncture and the Philosophy of the
Far East. Los Angeles: Tao Books, 1971.

Ohsawa, George. The Unique Principle. San Francisco:
Geo. Ohsawa Macrobiotic Foundations, Inc., 1973.

Outline of Chinese Acupuncture, An. Peking: Foreign
Languages Press, 1975.

Palos, Stephan. The Chinese Art of Healing. New York:
Bantam Books, 1972.

Saran, Steve. Body Messages (charts I and II).
Boulder, CO: Aslan Enterprises, 1979.

Saran, Steve. Reflexology (chart). Boulder, CO: Aslan
Enterprises, 1979.

Saran, Steve. The Unique Principle, (chart). Boulder,
CO: Aslan Enterprises, 1979.

Segarl, Maybelle, R.N., R.D., N.D., I.D. Reflexology.
North Hollywood, CA: Melvin Powers/Wilshire Book
Company, 1976.

Serizawa, Katsusuke, Prof., M.D. Massage, the Oriental
Method. San Francison: Japan Trading Co., 1972.

Serizawa, Katsusuke, Prof., M.D. Tsubo: Vital Points
for Oriental Therapy: San Francisco: Japan
Publications Trading Co., 1976.

Shultz, William. Shiatsu: Japanese Finger Pressure
Therapy. New York: Bell Publishing Co., 1976.

Silverstein, M.E., et al. Acupuncture and Moxibustion
(prepared by the Dept. of Health, Ho Pei Providence,
China). New York: Schocken Books, Inc., 1975.

Stiefvater, Dr. Eric H. What is Acupuncture? How Does
It Work? England: Health Science Press, 1971.

Teeguarden, Iona. Acupressure Way of Health: Jin Shin
Do. San Francisco: Japan Publications Trading Co.,
1978.

Thakkur, Chandrashekhar, Dr. Ayurveda: The Indian Art
and Science of Medicine. New York. ASI Publishers,
1974.

Thie, John F., D.C. Touch for Health. Santa Monica,
CA: DeVorss and Co., Publishers, 1973.

Tibetan Medicine. Berkeley, CA: University of
California Press, 1976.

Toguchi, Masaru. The Complete Guide to Acupuncture.
New York: Frederick Fell Publishers, Inc., 1974.

Veith, Ilza (translated and introduced by). The
Yellow Emperor's Classic of Internal Medicine (Huang
Ti Nei Ching Su Wen). Berkely, CA: University of
California Press, 1972.

Wallnofer, Heinrich, and Von Rottauscher, Anna.
Chinese Folk Medicine. New York: New American
Library, Inc., 1972.

Warren, Frank Z., M.D. Freedom From Pain Through
Acupressure. New York: Frederick Fell Publishers,
1976.

Wei-P'ing, Dr. Wu. Chinese Acupuncture. England:
Health Science Press, 1962.

Wilner, R. E., M.D. Acupuncture Desk Reference. North
Miami Beach, FL: Medical Diagnostic Institute, 1974.

Wilner, R. E., M.D. Confidential Report: Acupressure.
Miami Beach, FL: Medical Diagnostic Institute, 1979.

Yamamoto, Shizuko. Barefoot Shiatsu. San Francisco:
Japan Publications Trading Co., 1979.

Yanagiya, S. Prof., Dr. One-Needle Acupuncture.
London: The Acupuncture Association.